The Intermittent Fasting Impact for Woman

Unlock the hidden secrets to skyrocket fat loss & balance your hormones for those who hate diets

ISBN 978-0-6486577-4-3

Michael Zollo

Disclaimer Notice:

Please note the information contained within this document is for educational and entertainment purposes only. All effort has been executed to present accurate, up to date, and reliable, complete information. No warranties of any kind are declared or implied. Readers acknowledge that the author is not engaging in the rendering of legal, financial, medical or professional advice. The content within this book has been derived from various sources. Please consult a licensed professional before attempting any techniques outlined in this book.

By reading this document, the reader agrees that under no circumstances is the author responsible for any losses, direct or indirect, which are incurred as a result of the use of the information contained within this document, including, but not limited to, — errors, omissions, or inaccuracies. Always check with your medical professional before beginning any diet plan

The Intermittent Fasting Impact For Women

TABLE OF CONTENTS

From the author

I want to personally thank you for downloading my book *"The Intermittent Fasting Impact For Women."*

This book is exactly what the title suggests, a proven and time tested weight loss method that gets results. It got results 100 years ago, it gets results today and will continue to get results for people going forward.

It contains proven steps and strategies on how to use what I think is the most powerful weight loss tool out there, intermittent fasting makes losing weight absolutely effortless while being able to eat like a queen. It will keep you satisfied through your entire journey.

Before we get into that I would like to tell you a little about myself and my body transformation journey, i have been a personal trainer for over 10 years and have tried and tested many different approaches to weight loss. Although many of them worked initially, they all ended up being unsustainable and thus the end result was always the same, the weight would come back on and the yo-yo dieting method continued.

About 5 or so years into my personal training journey I ended up suffering from anxiety and small amounts of depression due to a few personal issues that were happening in my life at the time. As a result I did what so many other people do and I turned to food as my remedy.

Along with this, my training slowed down and became very up and down. Sometimes I would train 5 days per week then the next week only once. While my training slowed down my eating increased and the weight began to pile on along with more anxiety and more depression.

All of a sudden I wasn't looking so much like a personal trainer but more someone who needed a personal trainer. I ended up quitting and getting a desk job which I hated. So now not only was my activity level decreasing with my lack of gym work, I had also gone from a physical job as a PT to a sedentary job sitting at a desk yet my calorie intake was just as high if not higher than what they were when I was at my peak physical condition, not to mention the quality of the food was without a doubt worse.

Once again the weight took another spike and you guessed it, the result was more anxiety and more depression.

It wasn't until I was on vacation and saw a photo of myself without a shirt on that I was able to see just how out of shape I had become and how far I had let go of myself.

It was at that point that I made a promise to myself that

when I got back from vacation things were going to change. I got back into the gym training 5 days per week and began eating my 6 small meals a day every 3 hours to keep my metabolism "running high" as all mainstream fitness professionals recommend including myself at the time.

It lasted about 2 weeks and I fell of the wagon again. I was a different person to the one I was before and exercising 5 days a week was not sustainable anymore and since I was now working a regular desk job with a boss breathing down neck I wasn't able to stop and eat every 3 hours like I once did when I worked for myself as a PT.

I had to find another way.

I began looking into intermittent fasting and what it could do for me as far as helping me get back into shape. It's something I knew a little about already but never really researched it heavily because I had had it drummed into my head as a PT that not eating for more than 3 hours slowed down your metabolism and made you store fat. At this point in my life I was desperate, out of shape and had nothing to lose so I decided to give it a go.

I can tell you it was the best thing I have ever done as far as my health goes. Over the next year I began to transform my body in a way that I can only describe as effortless, it was both sustainable and effective. Yes of course I worked hard and I was consistent but the fact that I was able to enjoy some of the comfort foods I use to avoid years earlier along with being able to eat big satisfying meals that left me feeling full all while losing fat at the same time, made this method a game changer for me.

Along with this I decided to take more of a minimalist approach to my workouts as well. I decided I was going to do 3 gym sessions a week and then just add a light walk in between those sessions instead of the 5-6 workouts that use to take over my life at one stage.

My body felt great and I was literally doing half the work I was doing when I was a fully fledged fitness nut a few years earlier. I had hit the jackpot, a healthy body which I was happy with aesthetically, accompanied by a healthy mind and plenty of recovery time so I never burnt out and didn't feel like I had to live in a gym to maintain it.

Fitness should enhance your life not take away from it and working out 6 days a week as well as stopping every 3 hours to eat a small meal that never satisfied me took more from my life than it gave back. On top of this I would find myself in the middle of a decent binge eating session more often than I would have liked due to those small meals and cutting out the foods I love.

All I wanted was to find a way that I could still enjoy some of the foods that I loved most (not all of them healthy) while still being able to improve my body at the same time.

This is a weight loss system that SIMPLY WORKS, it is easy to follow and has many other health benefits other than the weight loss which I will cover throughout this book.

Below is my own personal before and after photos. I hope it inspires you to take action while you are reading through this book.

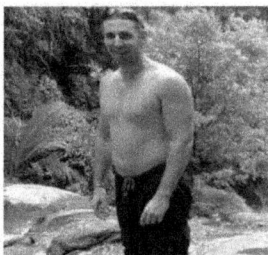

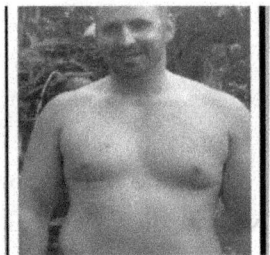

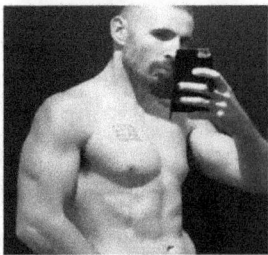

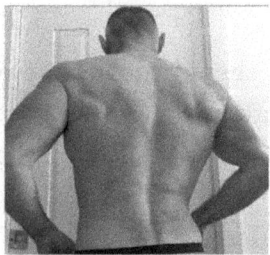

Free Report

As a thank you for purchasing this book I'd like to offer you a free report I have that goes into the top 8 trap foods that can destroy your road to a successful weight loss journey, most of which you probably see as healthy snack choices

On top of this I will tell you about the 4 popular diet tips you should NEVER follow.

Simply go to **www.vipfastingreport.com** and join my VIP community and I will send it to you instantly, it won't cost you a dime. On top of this you will also receive more advice, hacks and strategies to improve your health and well-being as well as discount offers exclusive only to my VIP community.

Also if you would like some extra support and want to surround yourself with other people working through the same struggles on the same journey as you are then join my free Facebook accountability group.

Just type in **effortless weight loss and functional strength** and be sure to answer the 3 questions and I will accept your request

Also follow me on Instagram at effortless_weightloss for more advice, motivation and advice.

If you have any questions feel free to reach out to me at **Michael.zollo@hotmail.com** I answer every email personally.

Introduction

Intermittent fasting is a practice that humanity has been using for thousands of years as a means of achieving a higher consciousness or for religious purposes. More recently, however, it has been gaining new converts thanks to its ability to help people lose weight while also letting them absorb a more significant amount of nutrients from the foods they eat than would otherwise be possible. People who participate in this new type of targeted intermittent fasting enjoy it because it doesn't require taking time out of your life every 3 hours to have a meal, nor does it require large amounts of time to prepare your food for the week.

The most basic form of intermittent fasting requires people to skip breakfast before going on to eat regularly throughout the rest of the day. This unrestrictive diet plan is a terrific choice for those who find sticking to traditional diet plans practically impossible as it requires fewer changes to your diet overall while still producing noticeable results almost from the start. Many users find success via intermittent fasting in both the short and the long-term because it is relatively easy to stick with once you get used to it while still providing results comparable to more traditional diet plans.

The reason that intermittent fasting is so useful comes

from the basic fact that the body behaves quite differently when it is in a fed state compared to when it is in a fasted state. A fed state is any period where the body is absorbing nutrients from foods it is actively digesting. This process begins roughly 5 minutes after you have finished a meal and lasts for about 5 hours depending on the type of foods you consumed as well as the quantity. While your body is being occupied by this process, it is also creating insulin which signals your body to store the food it has taken in as body fat or glycogen. During this time, it is impossible to burn fat as your body is in storage mode.

Once digestion has finished, the body enters a buffer period that can last up to 12 hours depending on what was eaten last and personal digestive differences. It takes the body this long to process the insulin that was created after the previous meal and get back to the level it started from. Only after these levels have once again normalized will your body be able to move back into a fasting state in which it can burn fat as efficiently as possible.

Chapter 1: What is Intermittent Fasting and Why Does It Work?

Intermittent Fasting (IF) may just be the best-kept secret in the diet and fitness industry, even though it may surprise you to learn that it has been practiced throughout the course of human history. With over 100 years of research to back up this fantastic game-changing lifestyle, intermittent fasting is poised to take the health and wellness community by storm.

Since 2010, the number of online searches for "intermittent fasting" has increased by more than 9,000 percent, with the majority of this increase happening within the last few years. With this renewed surge in popularity, intermittent fasting is quickly becoming a hot new alternative that many people are turning to for a wide variety of reasons not limited to weight loss and transformation.

Before we jump into what intermittent fasting is, and why it works, let's first go over a couple of things that intermittent fasting is not.

First, intermittent fasting is NOT a diet plan. There are no off-limit foods, no meal plans, no meal prepping, and no complicated recipes. In fact, you can practice intermittent fasting and eat whatever you want. You'll still get some of the benefits. Of course, occasional fasting works the best when you try to eat more vegetables and whole foods while eating less processed foods. However, it isn't necessary, and you can keep having treats without any guilt.

Second, intermittent fasting is NOT a metabolism lowering calorie restriction game. In fact, occasional fasting can be used to lose weight, maintain weight, or even gain muscle. What does this mean for you? If you like intermittent fasting, and it ends up being a good fit, you can practice it for the rest of your life. Of course it helps you lose weight, but it has so many more benefits that go along with that.

Intermittent Fasting: The Basics

Let's get down to it. What is intermittent fasting? In short, intermittent fasting is a pattern of eating that involves periods of starvation, and periods of feasting. If this sounds frightening, don't worry! You've already been practicing the traditional eating pattern for your whole life.

This is what you've probably been taught: breakfast is the most important meal of the day, and you need to eat it about 30 minutes to 1 hour after you wake up. Your day should consist of three large meals and two snacks. Many of us, especially those following the Standard

American Diet (SAD), have been taught to believe this eating pattern is best for our health. This is an old school, out dated method.

But what if there was a body of research out there that proved otherwise? What if I told you that by not eating for periods of 16, 24, or even 36 hours, you could lose weight, gain muscle, boost your energy levels and overall health? Well, this is all true, and it's called intermittent fasting.

There are several different methods of intermittent fasting, and you will learn how to incorporate the top four in a later chapter. For now, let's just go over the basics. To practice intermittent fasting, you don't eat for 16+ hours. For most people, that means eating dinner at 7pm, going to sleep, and then not eating again until lunch the next day. Not eating for 16 hours might sound hard, but it becomes a lot easier if you sleep through 8 of those hours!

Like many people, you may already have practiced intermittent fasting without realizing it. Let's take a second and consider the aforementioned term "breakfast", or better yet, "break-fast". This word refers to the meal that "breaks" your "fast". Going to bed after eating and waking up the next morning for your first meal of the day has already constituted a period of fasting, even if it is only for a short duration. Never been a breakfast person? No problem! If you have ever woken up late on the weekend, or met a friend for a late brunch around noon, and that is your first meal of the day, you have already practiced intermittent fasting.

If your first reaction to this is reluctance, keep reading. Over the next chapters, we will discuss why intermittent fasting is the right lifestyle for you and how you can easily integrate it into your life. Now, you may think to yourself; I'll be so hungry if I skip breakfast! We'll get more into this later, but after the first week or two, you really won't feel hungry! Your mind is used to eating in the morning, so for the first week, you will feel hungry. Once your brain learns to wait until lunch for food that hunger will go away. In many ways, intermittent fasting teaches you to listen to your body more closely.

Why Intermittent Fasting? - Basic Bonuses

So why choose intermittent fasting? Before we dive into all the specific health benefits, let's take a quick look at some of the basic reasons why intermittent fasting may be a good alternative for you.

- You don't have to be a rocket scientist to figure out that not all calories are created equal, but the one important thing to always keep in mind is that they do play a crucial role in weight and fat loss (specifically by the process of caloric restriction). When you fast, you make it easier to limit your total caloric intake since you are physically limiting the amount of time that you have to eat. By doing this, you can expect to see consistent weight loss and/or maintenance that can better help you achieve your goals. Pretty easy, right.

- Another great reason why intermittent fasting can be a good option is that it can help simplify your day. Living in the 21st century (well at least physically, maybe not mentally), pretty much everything revolves around an "on-the-go" lifestyle with hardly any time for ourselves. How then can we expect to follow strict diets that require specific recipes, meal prepping, and even a scheduled table of eating times? Well, don't worry, with intermittent fasting you don't have to. Intermittent fasting allows you to simply skip a meal or two and only ever have to worry about eating food within your "eating window". Just one less decision and task you have to worry about making every day.

- If we stick with the same theme (no crazy diets), intermittent fasting can also allow you to enjoy larger meals. Rather than leave your taste buds and stomach high and dry, with intermittent fasting you can still enjoy large meals that give you a feeling of satisfaction. Did we also mention that by doing this you can still, on average, eat fewer calories in a day? Many other diets and fads limit your caloric intake, but at a price - the feeling of hunger after every meal.

- Finally, a major component of intermittent fasting, especially for those of us with busy lifestyles, is that IF can require significantly less time (and in some cases, less money) to achieve. Rather than having to prepare and prep meals for each upcoming day, or even worse, purchase four to six meals a day, intermittent fasting can help reduce the number of meals you need, saving you valuable time and, depending on some factors, the money in your wallet as well!

Less meals? What about binge eating?

Since intermittent fasting requires longer periods of time without eating, it may also seem like sometimes you are overcompensating for the lack of meals by overeating when you decide to break your fast. While this has been the pervading thought for quite some time, there are many studies that indicate that overcompensating for skipping a meal is simply a myth.

While you will certainly eat more at your meal times when you break your fast, it still isn't enough to make up for an entire meal that you missed - hence the beauty and advantage of intermittent fasting! While it may feel as if you are over-consuming and eating too much, often times you are in fact eating less due to not only the decrease in the amount of meals, but also because your body can only handle so much until it decides its full. Once you have reached this level you no longer feel the desire to eat. Pair this with the aforementioned point of less meals, and you are still eating less calories than you may otherwise do with 4-6 regularly spaced out meals.

But what if you are still worried about binge eating? Or even worse, find yourself actually struggling with it. Don't worry! For those of you concerned with binge eating when trying to follow intermittent fasting (or already following it), there are some key steps you can take.

1. **Did you consume enough the day before?**

   If you feel like you are binging and eating too much when you break your fast, stop and ask yourself if you have managed to get enough calories in your body to keep it going. Often times this can be a result of under-eating or a shortage in the number of calories you have consumed the previous day. If you find yourself struggling with this, or think it is the problem, try tracking your food and calorie intake for a week or so to see what is going on. Tracking your food intake can be a great way of not only better understanding your eating habits and how they affect you, but also improve your knowledge and understanding about the food itself.

2. **Check your foods, are they nutrient dense?**

   When you start cooking from scratch and using fresh ingredients you can really begin to see why you don't need to eat every hour. Using this method can give you a first-hand look at how proper food consumption can nourish your body and give you the energy and feeling of well-being that you need.

Starting intermittent fasting without taking a good, hard look at the food you are putting into your body can cause serious problems and implications down the road, especially in the case of binge eating. Intermittent fasting is not a magic pill that fixes everything. On the contrary, you need to be eating nutrient rich and nutrient dense food in order to succeed and stay on track. Not only can these foods help give you the energy that you need, but they can also help alleviate a feeling of emptiness when trying to go long periods of time without eating.

3. Maybe you have bitten off more than you can chew? (no pun intended)

If you are a newbie just starting to think about intermittent fasting, or even someone who has tried it, but failed, take a second and think about the best option for yourself. Intermittent fasting can be tough, especially if you decide to jump right into a straight 16 hour fast. If you find yourself thinking this may be a reason, maybe you have taken on too much too soon?

When using intermittent fasting, play around with how long you are fasting for. Of course, anything over 12 hours is going to have great fat loss opportunities and health benefits, but

DON'T FORCE IT. It is important to ease your body into the process and get a feel for what it is like and what you are doing. This can be extremely helpful in aiding any binge eating that might occur due to the unexpected and unanticipated challenges between prolonged periods of not eating.

4. Is eating just one or two meals right for everyone?

If you find yourself thinking that you feel like you are doing everything right, but still binge eating, then maybe the answer might simply be that one to two meals per day just isn't the right thing for you personally.

But wait! Don't abandon hope in intermittent fasting just yet! Even if you find yourself in this predicament, it doesn't mean that you can't get the fat loss and health benefits from following an intermittent fasting plan. Instead, it just means that maybe you need/should eat three or four smaller meals rather than just the larger one to two meals during your "eating window". You can still aim for your designated fasting period every day, but you will just be consuming your calories in a different way that better suits your needs.

Having discussed a few key steps in helping to alleviate binge eating, or more importantly, preventing it, we can now see that there are many ways in which we can make intermittent fasting work for us. Everyone has a different relationship with food and meal times. What works for one person does not necessarily mean it will work for someone else.

Intermittent fasting can be a very personal, and in some cases, challenging, journey. Not only can it take more than a few days to become a lean, mean, fat burning machine, but it can also take a lot longer to find and decide upon the best and most effective method for you! When beginning or using intermittent fasting, remember, it's quite okay to play around with meal frequency, food type, and the length of fasting time. In fact I recommend that you do. Trial and error is the best way to come up with your perfect method of fasting, try things see what works, see what doesn't and adjust as you go.

Intermittent Fasting and Your Body's Chemistry

Insulin tells our body when it is time to store energy as fat, and when it is time to burn fat as energy. When we eat, our stomach and liver turn food into energy. Some of that power goes into our bloodstream as blood sugar, and we use that immediately. The rest? Stored as fat.

Insulin is a chemical, that is released by our pancreas when we eat, it tells our body it is time to store fat. So when we don't eat for 16 hours or more, our insulin levels go down significantly, and our body transitions into fat burning mode. Thus, even if you ate a large dinner the night before, you'll still go into fat burning mode the next morning!

Insulin isn't the only chemical that a fast triggers, however. When we fast for longer than 16 hours, our body produces more human growth hormone (HGH). This artificial hormone tells our body to burn fat, repair muscle, and even build new muscles! By fasting, you will lose weight and have more energy!

If this isn't enough well there is one more reason that intermittent fasting kicks the 6 small meals a day weight loss plan: when you fast for over 16 hours, your body produces more adrenaline. Adrenaline, in turn, gives you more energy and mental awareness! You'll feel energetic and thoughtful even when you haven't eaten for a long period of time.

The combination of these three effects, lower insulin, increased HGH, and increased adrenaline, combine in your body to raise your metabolism, sometimes up to 14% higher than your base rate. You will also be reducing your calories somewhat since you eat fewer meals each day. This slight calorie reduction, plus increased metabolism, will lead to fantastic and long-lasting results both on the outside aesthetically and on the inside with your overall health.

Chapter 2: The Health Benefits of Intermittent Fasting

Do you have a complicated medical history in your family? Are you overweight? Maybe you're nervous about diabetes, obesity, or heart disease. The fact is, when the body is in fasting mode, you release hormones that tell the cells in your body that it is time to take action. Once triggered, these cells can help aid the body in many of the necessary functions to resolve the issue(s) and can even help eliminate many of the first signs of disease. By practicing intermittent fasting, we give our batteries more time to heal, providing ourselves with increased longevity in our lives.

Intermittent Fasting for Weight Loss

Intermittent fasting allows the body to utilize its stored energy in order to help burn off excess body fat, helping lead to additional benefits such as overall weight loss and better body composition.

Before we dive right in to the how and why of this, it is important to realize that fasting is in fact a normal and natural process of the body. Contrary to what you may believe, throughout history, we as humans have actually evolved and developed to fast for shorter periods of time (hours or days, instead of days or weeks).

Jetting back through time and space for a moment, consider the days of the caveman. How did they survive? What was life like for them on a daily basis? One thing is for sure, there were no supermarkets, fast food restaurants, or 24-hour convenience stores. The food our primordial ancestors ate was simply what they had available - what could be scavenged for, hunted for, or maybe even grown. If nothing was available, they didn't eat, but when the times got tough, what exactly allowed them to survive?

Before all the luxuries of modern-day society, fasting for longer periods of time was in fact quite normal. The truth of the matter is that the body is actually built to function in a way which will allow it to do everything it possibly can to preserve and sustain itself for as long as possible. But how you ask? Well, one reason is by storing fat.

Our body's produce and store body fat (sometimes in the places we don't want it of course) for a later date. Since body fat is simply the energy from food stored away, if you do not eat (or can't eat), your body realizes this and simply "eats" its own saved fat for energy.

When we eat, more food energy is immediately ingested that can be used by our bodies at that exact time. While there are a plethora of other factors that determine how much food energy will be stored overall, our body is designed so that no matter what, some of the energy will be immediately saved and stockpiled away for a later time - like a futuristic defense mechanism. The reason for this is that the body cannot predict when its next food source will be or how long it may have to go before being replenished. By storing excess food energy, the body is essentially creating a "reserve pack" of additional energy for the unforeseen future.

So how does this happen?

When we eat, the insulin (a key contributing hormone) in our body helps to break down and store the surplus energy. Carbohydrates (a favorite indulgence of many) especially, are broken down into individual glucose (sugar) units which are then transformed into long chains which form glycogen. These molecules are then stored in the liver or muscles for later use. While this is a great first step, there is however very limited storage space for carbohydrates. Once the maximum capacity is reached, the liver then starts to kick in and turn the excess glucose into fat through a process known as "de-novo lipogenesis" - the making of new fat.

While some of this newly created fat will get stored onsite in the liver, for the most part, the majority of it will be transported to other fat deposit and "storage" areas in the body. While this is a much more complicated process, which we won't go into detail about here, the important thing to comprehend is that there is pretty much no set limit to the amount of additional fat that can be created and thus looking for a new home.

So, what exactly does all this mean? Well, as more and more fat is created, it must be stored somewhere in the body. Unfortunately for us, it is often stored in the areas of the body that everyone despises such as love handles, lower belly, hips, etc.

So how does intermittent fasting help us alleviate this problem?

When we don't eat, the process we just highlighted above, inverts itself. When there is no food available, insulin levels fall, triggering a response in the body to start burning its stored energy reserves since there is nothing coming through to provide the energy.

When we compile all this information together, we can see that the body really only exists in two states: 1) the fed state (characterized by high insulin levels) and 2) the fasted state (determined by relatively low or lower insulin levels).

Depending on what we choose to do (eating or fasting), our bodies are either storing food energy (adding to our reserves) or burning stored energy (tapping into and decreasing our reserves), its one or the other, not both. If our eating and fasting are balanced, then typically there should be no changes in weight as everything is in perfect harmony. If they are not balanced, then we can expect to see effects stemming from whichever side the scale is tipped - fat/weight loss or fat/weight gain.

In a nutshell, intermittent fasting allows the body to use and consume its own stored energy. The important thing to keep in mind and understand is that there is nothing wrong with doing this, it is what our body is designed to do and how is is designed to function.

If you are always eating every third to fourth hour (as is often recommended or advised), then your body may constantly use the incoming food for energy and may not need to break down and burn much body fat - if any at all. You may just be storing fat, saving it for a time when your body anticipates that there will be nothing to eat. If this happens to you, then using intermittent fasting may be a beneficial and conducive way to help you resolve the problem and get rid of that extra body fat.

Intermittent Fasting for Stress and Inflammation

While inflammation is not always a bad kind of bodily response, it is still something that should be monitored and controlled as much as possible. Our body experiences inflammation when we are trying to heal ourselves and recover from strenuous activity or injury, but when the inflammation lasts for prolonged periods of time there is a significant risk of negative impacts on our health.

Stress and inflammation are two of the major contributors and advances towards aging and many other chronic diseases (including such things as gastrointestinal diseases, arthritis, obesity, asthma, and even cancer).

Oxidative stress involves unstable molecules, often referred to as "free radicals", which interact with other very important molecules (like DNA, protein, etc.) and cause significant damage to them. When these molecules become damaged or unable to be eliminated by the body it can lead to higher levels of inflammation or even chronic inflammation. In addition to the aforementioned problems, having higher or chronic levels of inflammation can lead to further complications such as back pain, arthritis, and osteoporosis.

While this may sound more alarming than you originally thought, don't panic! Recent studies have actually found a positive correlation and impact between fasting and chronic inflammation. It is believed that intermittent fasting may help and assist in managing stress and inflammation by changing how compounds and proteins transact with one another and thus inhibit inflammatory pathways and reducing or possibly eliminating the problem all together.

Do you have a complicated medical history in your family? Maybe you're nervous about diabetes, or heart disease. The fact is, when the body is in fasting mode, you release hormones that tell the cells in your body that it is time to go into repair mode. In this repair mode, the cells can eliminate many of the first signs of disease. By practicing intermittent fasting, we give our batteries more time to heal, providing ourselves with increased longevity in our lives.

Intermittent Fasting and Diabetes

The first health benefit to come from intermittent fasting originates with that little, fat regulating chemical, insulin. Insulin is probably most famous for its role in causing or preventing the onset of diabetes.

Today, diabetes is not the debilitating disease it once

was, as long as it is caught early and dealt with responsibly. In fact, most people don't need to suffer from diabetes. Adding intermittent fasting to your lifestyle can help prevent the onset of type 2 diabetes.

This is because type 2 diabetes is the form of the disease that is mostly triggered by an unhealthy diet and lifestyle. The body develops insulin resistance and therefore cannot regulate the amount of sugar in the bloodstream.

When we practice intermittent fasting, the body lowers its overall insulin level. Periods of low insulin helps prevent against insulin resistance. In one study conducted on human subjects, blood sugar was reduced up to 6% during a fast.

A further study conducted on rats with diabetes showed that intermittent fasting helped prevent and protect the kidney from damage. This has not yet been tested in humans.

Okay, so intermittent fasting helps prevent diabetes. But what if diabetes isn't a concern for you? No one in your family has ever had diabetes, and your diet right now isn't that bad. Okay, fine. What about a much more common and more deadly disease? What about cancer?

Intermittent Fasting and Cancer

It's true; intermittent fasting can help prevent and protect the body from developing certain cancers. How? Let's find out.

First of all, intermittent fasting can reduce oxidative stress and inflammation in the body. Oxidative stress is a fancy way of talking about the cell's natural ability to detoxify itself. If this process of detoxification is interrupted or blocked, oxidative stress occurs. Unfortunately, eating a bad diet, or overeating, can lead to increased oxidative stress and inflammation in the body. These two things can lead to cancer.

There have been a few studies that illustrate the relationship between intermittent fasting and reduced oxidative stress and inflammation. If you're trying to prevent or even heal a chronic disease, or cancer, intermittent fasting could be an excellent choice for you.

So what if you, or someone you love, already have cancer? Based on a study done on human patients, there is some evidence that intermittent fasting can help reduce some of the side effects of chemotherapy!

Probably the most crucial benefit of intermittent fasting is its ability to trigger autophagy in the cells. What is autophagy? It's a fancy way of saying "repair mode." When we are eating every three hours, cells are continuously reproducing, using the new food to create new cells. When we pause and enter a short fasting period, the cells shift into repair mode.

This repair mode, known as autophagy, is essential for healthy cellular life in our bodies. Increasing the amount of repair in our bodies can protect us against certain diseases, including cancer, and Alzheimer's.

Intermittent Fasting and the Brain

Yes, that's right, intermittent fasting can even help prevent Alzheimer's. The research on this claim is still rudimentary, but preliminary studies on rats show that intermittent fasting may delay or slow the onset of Alzheimer's. We need more research on human studies before we can make any bolder claims than that, but for now, better safe than sorry, right?

Even if Alzheimer's isn't a concern for you, there are many more benefits to the brain from intermittent fasting? The boost that IF gives to your metabolism also impacts your brain function.

Studies in animals have shown that intermittent fasting reduces brain damage, strokes, and improves mental functioning over time. I know personally the most productive part of my day comes during my fast, especially when I add a little black coffee into the equation (black coffee on its own of course as adding any fillers will immediately break your fast), I feel awake, alert and have a high level of mental focus that I certainly don't get directly after a meal.

Intermittent Fasting and the Heart

You may think we are done here. There can't be ANY more health benefits, right? Wrong. There is one more significant health benefit to be earned from a lifestyle of intermittent fasting: lowered risk of heart disease.

Today in America, heart disease is a killer. It is one of the leading causes of death among adults, especially among adults struggling with obesity or weight gain.

Good news for American adults. Intermittent fasting has been shown, in animal studies, to improve on many different risk factors related to heart disease. It reduces blood pressure, cholesterol levels, blood triglycerides, inflammation, and blood sugar levels. There can't be a better lifestyle choice out there where heart health is concerned.

Yes, this all sounds too good to be true. A simple lifestyle change such as not eating for 16 hours can lead to all of these benefits? Increased health, weight loss, along with heightened energy and mental alertness? It seems impossible. There must be a catch. It must lead to binge eating because you'll be so hungry after the fast!

Intermittent Fasting and Life Longevity

One exciting and advantageous possibility of intermittent fasting may be its effectiveness in helping to extend lifespan!

According to some experts, a vital aspect of fasting, unrelated to simple calorie restriction, is that the body undergoes a metabolic switch from using glucose as the primary source of fuel to using ketones. You may have heard that term from the latest diet craze, the Keto diet Since we know that the body will either burn sugar or fat for energy, when blood sugar levels drop and glycogen stores are used up, the body begins to use ketones for energy.

The presence of ketones in the blood can help signify that the body, on a cellular level, is trying to "regenerate" itself, which can help protect against disease and aging. By altering the activity of the mitochondrial networks inside our cells, restricted diets like intermittent fasting can help promote better homeostasis in mitochondrial networks allowing for a healthier and more adequate response time to metabolic alteration to meet our body's needs.

To sum it up, when you stop eating or perform a fast, you increase your body's "mitochondrial energy efficiency". Not only does this help your body burn fat as an energy source, but also increases overall health on the cellular level - a key component in aiding longevity.

Chapter 3: The Overall Benefits of Intermittent Fasting

Intermittent fasting has helped many people lose weight and become the best versions of them. This pattern of eating is not a short-term diet, but a long-term lifestyle. Why? Because it has a whole list of research-backed health benefits that go way beyond weight loss.

Mental Benefits

- Improved metabolism, which is beneficial to Brain Health, Metabolism is the name for the essential chemical reactions that happen in your cells. We talk about having a fast or slow metabolism all the time without really understanding how vital it is to the conversion of food to fuel and composing the building blocks for proteins and carbohydrates and the elimination of cellular waste.
- Improved Ketone production. Ketone is a chemical that protects the brain when there is a decrease of available glucose.
- May reduce symptoms of depression by regulating insulin and blood sugar levels.
- Enhances performance on memory tests in the elderly
- May play a preventative role in those suffering

from anxiety through regulation of glucose and decreased oxidative stress. As stated earlier oxidative stress happens when the body can't detox the harmful effects of free radicals (uncharged molecules) fast enough.

Systemic Benefits

- Cellular Repair – through autophagy, which is given more focus in a FASTING State.
- Hormonal Rebalancing – Insulin Levels and Insulin Resistance; Leptin; Ghrelin and Human Growth Hormone increases and facilitates fat burning and muscle gain
- Gene protection – Related to longevity and protection against diseases, including promising research on cancer
- Reduces Oxidative stress, damage, and inflammation in the body

Quality of Life Benefits

- May improve sleep patterns – If your intermittent fasting schedule includes eating a meal 3 to 4 hours before sleeping and contains carbohydrates, your sleep quality and quantity could grow due to increased production of serotonin, a chemical in the body that helps regulate cyclic body processes, such as the sleep cycle, as well as contributing to feelings of happiness and wellbeing. I eat my last meal of the day right before bed and the quality of my sleep as improved dramatically compared to when I use to stop eating carbs 6 hours before bed.

- Increased stamina – Athletes who exercise on an empty stomach have experienced more energy and strength. It is believed that the combination of fasting and exercising triggers internal catalysts that force the breakdown of sugars and fat into power, without sacrificing muscle mass. This is a claim that a lot of bodybuilders and old school fitness professional would strongly disagree with. I have lived a lifestyle of eating every 3 hours prior to implementing fasting into my life and I can honestly say that aesthetically muscle to fat ratio I am in the best condition of my life as a 37 year old. I can also report that my energy levels for my workout have not suffered either, it's a win/win situation from where I sit.

Behavioral Benefits

- Improves appetite control – Intermittent Fasting allows you to understand the difference between mental and physical hunger
- Helps with food cravings – As your Leptin and Ghrelin levels reset to your intermittent fasting schedule, old triggers that caused you to eat

certain foods at certain times will be erased. Also, periodic fasting doesn't ban specific foods; only the period in which you can consume them!

- Develops an appreciation for high-quality food—when you learn to eat within a specific time frame and fast through another, you learn to appreciate the gift of eating good quality food. You may notice that you savor food more, eating it slower as well as having a much keener sense of when you are becoming full. You will also discover certain high-quality food sources such as whey protein, green vegetables and berries are ingested and incorporated faster into your system, due to their nutritionally dense makeup. This also makes them perfect post workout foods.

Fiscal and Timesaving Benefits

- Save money – Depending on your intermittent fasting schedule, you could end up skipping seven meals or more a week. As long as you don't add the caloric total of these meals to the meals you DO consume then could cutting up to a day's worth of food out of your budget. Take a page from the Mormon faith and add up how much money and time you save by not purchasing and preparing these meals. Whether you pay that savings forward or keep it for a rainy day is up to you!

- Save time – This particular benefit personally resonates with me. As a former dieter, I can say with the voice of an expert, that many of the miracle diets and fads I have tried in my quest to lose weight not only included a lot of really expensive ingredients but also took hours away from my life to prepare. Hours that I would never get back and hours that were best spent doing other things I enjoyed doing ahead of cooking. When you choose to fast intermittently, you automatically save a certain percentage of weekly food prep basically because you SKIP the entire process. It's up to you how ugly or fancy your remaining meals are. The important thing is to eat a balanced, clean, nutritious menu of food and if you overindulge a day or two on vacation or out with friends on a Saturday night? Well then tomorrow is another day so don't stress over it.

Personal Growth Benefits

- Taking on a physical and mental challenge and being rewarded with the ability to balance health and nutritional needs.
- Acquiring an excellent tool for strength training or other athletic challenges.
- Experiencing consistent, balanced control over essential life choices.
- Gaining the flexibility and freedom to choose

when you eat socially with friends and family, and when you take a planned break.

- Experiencing Mind/Body connection in a visceral manner that regulates when, why and how you eat.
- Learning how to be mindful when eating
- Experiencing delayed gratification rather than immediate gratification
- Developing resilience in a controlled setting
- Learning how to respect boundaries and how to be nutritionally creative within them

As I hope you can see the diverse spectrum of benefits I've included above, I believe that the practice of Intermittent Fasting offers you much, much more than a diet. As I've stated before, it's an important, valuable life choice – the rewards that will be gained from incorporating it into your health regime and lifestyle can easily be transferred into many other parts of your life. I am a big advocate of connecting mind, body and spirit into a cohesive, healthy, balanced unit, transforming us all into empowered individuals; ready to take on all the opportunities this world has to offer!

Chapter 4: Intermittent Fasting for Women

Specific Effects of Intermittent Fasting on the Female Body And Precautions For Potential Hazards

In the previous two chapters we explained exactly what intermittent fasting is, as well as some of the benefits you can expect to experience while following this dietary lifestyle. While the effects that we discussed are the same for both men and women, this chapter is about intermittent fasting for women. Therefore, we will focus on the effects of intermittent fasting more specific to the female body. Furthermore, while there are a plethora of benefits that women can reap from choosing to fast, there are also some health concerns unique to women that we should discuss, as well as how you can avoid them. After all, if you choose to begin intermittent fasting to live a healthier and fuller life, the last thing you want is to create new health problems in the process!

We have discussed how intermittent fasting can help both men and women lose weight, have more energy, and even lower their risk for various types of disease. However, there have been numerous studies performed using only women as subjects where intermittent fasting has proven to be extremely effective at providing these benefits. A study published in the International Journal of Obesity in 2011 selected two groups of women and subjected them to two different methods of fasting, continuous (no food for an entire day) and intermittent. While both groups of women lost weight, the group that adhered to intermittent fasting saw 30% of the women lose anywhere from 5-10% of their body weight, and 34% of these women lost over 10% of their body weight.

What is even more remarkable about these findings is that these women were not instructed to exercise, and made little if any changes in their amount of physical activity during this study! We are not talking about a few pounds here and there, without even taking exercise into consideration, these women were able to lose a remarkable amount of body weight by just trying intermittent fasting. While this study was performed to see how fasting has impacted weight loss in women, researchers also wanted to see if this lifestyle was really effective in preventing certain diseases. They measured certain risk markers for things such as diabetes, cancer, and cardiovascular disease in these women before the study began, and immediately afterwards. What they found was that after following the intermittent fasting protocol, these risk markers were decreased substantially in all of the women.

Another study published in the Nutrition Journal in 2012 aimed to learn what happened to the energy needs in the female body when fasting begins. A group of women were selected to follow an 8-week, calorically restricted intermittent fasting plan. What they found was that these women actually had a huge reduction in their body's energy needs, between 75-90%! Intermittent fasting makes the female body incredibly more efficient and teaches it to use energy much more effectively. Once again, the human body is an incredible piece of machinery, and is extremely adaptive, it knows how to maintain itself at all costs. When it experiences fasting, it will teach itself to run just as well, if not better on fewer calories as it plunges into fat reserves to continue functioning optimally.

Now there are a few health concerns specific to the female body that I would like to address when it comes to intermittent fasting. The first of these are drastic hormonal food cravings. We touched on this subject earlier, but there are numerous hormones in the body that regulate and control hunger. These include insulin, leptin, and ghrelin, among many others. Women subjected to extended periods of fasting (as in not eating for an entire day) are susceptible to having these hormones thrown out of whack.

When this happens, the chemical signals in the brain that let you know when you are full and should not eat anymore actually turn off, which can cause overeating.

A study consisting of female college students at the University of Virginia had their subjects fast for two whole days. What they found was that levels of leptin in these women decreased by as much as 75%! This can severely disrupt feelings of satiety and result in someone consuming too many calories when the fasting period is over. The women in this study also experienced a 50% increase in their cortisol levels. Cortisol is more commonly referred to as the stress hormone.

Cortisol becomes elevated when we are worn out, nervous, afraid, and/or hungry. It can also cause us to crave sugary and fatty foods to try and feed our body a quick burst of highly available energy. The body craves this quick fix in order to deal with whatever short term situation we are in. This is simply another one of the body's survival mechanisms. As a woman, if you are following intermittent fasting to lose weight, the last thing you want is your cortisol level through the roof, begging you to eat that candy bar or drink a soda! So how can you avoid these hormonal cravings causing you to overeat and desire junk food? Well, instead of going on an extended fast such as 24 to 48 hours, you will simply narrow your food intake into an 8-10 hour feeding window, you can reap the benefits of intermittent fasting while burning fat and increasing your insulin sensitivity without throwing your hunger hormones for a loop.

Another serious side effect of intermittent fasting

unique to the female body is a disrupted menstrual cycle and even a decrease in ovary size. A study conducted using female rats found that after two weeks of intermittent fasting, the rat's menstrual cycles ceased completely and their ovaries were severely diminished. This is thought to be yet another survival mechanism in the mammalian body, it sort of makes sense if you think about it. If the female body believes that it is starving, and is trying to use as little energy available as efficiently possible, the last thing that needs to be introduced into the equation is a growing fetus that requires an enormous amount of energy to develop.

If a woman's body believes it is having a hard enough time keeping itself alive, Mother Nature will make some changes, such as bringing ovulation to a halt and shrinking their ovaries. This is to ensure that there will only be one human to keep alive for the time being. While this is a remarkable mechanism of survival that probably served our ancient ancestors well, you are not actually starving, and you most likely do not want to have your reproductive system thrown out of balance. So if you begin intermittent fasting and notice changes in your menstrual cycle and ovulation frequency, what can you do? Dr. Amy Shah, an expert of intermittent fasting protocols and their effects on the female anatomy recommends what she calls crescendo fasting.

What this entails is that women do not actually fast everyday, but select two to three days out of the week, preferably non-consecutive days such as Monday, Wednesday, and Friday, and on those days they will fast the usual 12-16 hours. On the days you are fasting, this method recommends women only engage in physical exercise such a light yoga, while saving any high intensity workouts for non-fasting days. After following this method for 2-3 weeks, women are encouraged to try and add one more fasting day during the week, and monitor their body's reaction. By partaking in crescendo fasting, women are more likely to see the benefits of intermittent fasting without their hormones and reproductive system going into all out panic mode.

While we are on the topic of possible disruptions to the female reproductive system, we will discuss a rather odd side effect that some women may possibly experience from intermittent fasting. The female body contains many unique biological mechanisms that are used specifically to aid in pregnancy and ensure the health of a fetus. Unfortunately, but also incredibly admirable, the female body is designed so that in times of hardship, such as starvation, the fetus will survive no matter the costs to the mother.

When resources and nutrition are running low, a growing fetus can actually cause hormonal changes in the female body to reroute vital nutrients to itself. Often when women are following any sort of fasting protocol, they experience severe, insatiable hunger when they break their fast. This is the way the female body protects a potential fetus, regardless if there is one or there's not. Because the female body is so uniquely designed to develop and nourish a growing baby, it will actually do whatever it takes to maintain an internal environment conducive to a baby's growth, even if there isn't one there!

To mitigate effects such as this one, experts recommend that women go for several trial fasts before diving headfirst into intermittent fasting. This can be done by consuming all food in an 8-hour feeding window maybe once a week, seeing how your body responds to it, and then adding a day if things go smoothly. However, if you choose to try out fasting, the key is to be gentle. The last thing you want is to begin an intense fasting regimen and make your body think famine has come and all will be lost if it doesn't protect your growing bundle of joy that isn't actually there. So, if you choose to begin intermittent fasting, it's always best to ease into it and the benefits will follow suit.

Another hormonal issue that women need to consider when beginning intermittent fasting, is their estrogen levels. While the male and female bodies both contain estrogen as well as testosterone, we all know that males contain much more testosterone than women, and women more estrogen than men. These hormones work to provide certain physical and emotional aspects that are unique to the different genders.

Estrogen, the primary female sex hormone, can actually make it harder or easier for a woman to stick with any dietary plan, especially intermittent fasting. The different craving levels will change depending on certain periods of the menstrual cycle throughout the month. The reason for this is because the hormone estrogen actually decreases appetite by reducing a woman's sensitivity to feeding cues, causing you to feel hungry less often. At certain periods in the menstrual cycle, such as the preovulatory phase, food intake is at its lowest. Likewise, during later periods in the menstrual cycle such as the follicular and luteal phases, food intake is actually increased.

But what does this mean for you? Well, assuming that you plan to adhere to intermittent fasting as a lifestyle, you are likely to have certain periods of the month when it just seems harder to stick to your feeding window. You may think you are just not exercising enough self-control, or that you are slacking in your commitment to eating healthier at these times, when really you are just the victim of a hormonal fluctuation that's out of your control. While there is no way to stop the fluctuation of estrogen in your body, (none that you want to try anyway) you can mitigate the intense hunger cravings in the same way that we've talked about reducing or preventing other unwanted side effects. Exercise moderation with intermittent fasting, especially when you first begin this lifestyle. As a female, your body is extremely sensitive to hormonal alterations and is likely to respond adversely if you go from your normal eating routine straight into a prolonged fast.

Although this chapter may seem to have portrayed intermittent fasting in a negative light, the hazards that we have discussed are all easily avoidable. As a woman, your body is designed to protect not only you, but also another human life growing inside of you through the body's delicate hormone balance and biological mechanisms. As long as you approach intermittent fasting from a reasonable perspective with this new found awareness, I truly believe that you can experience the many benefits available from this lifestyle, without falling victim to the possible negative side effects I have mentioned.

Remember that moderation is key when starting this protocol. The body is extremely intelligent at sensing small changes or fluctuations in your internal and external environments. The body likes to stay in its comfort zone, it hates change and will turn to drastic measures to protect itself and maintain homeostasis. Therefore, when beginning any sort of new diet or exercise program, you should always gradually implement the change into your day-to-day life rather than going from one extreme to another.

You would never attempt to run a marathon without starting a progressive training program. Maybe running a mile every day until that became easy, and then moving on to running half-marathons, etc. The same logic applies to intermittent fasting. It's not a good idea to go from eating your normal breakfast, lunch, and dinner with a snack in between, then suddenly go 16 hours without eating.

You know when you see those commercials play on television advertising a type of medicine? Then at the end of the ad an unnecessarily fast speaker chimes in to list off about 50 possible side effects listed in the fine print at the bottom of your screen? Although the side effects they mention only occur in a very small percentage of individuals that take the medicine, they still have to inform you of them for your health and safety. This chapter serves to delve into that purpose and thoroughly explain any of the female issues that could possibly arrive, so you are aware of them and know how to avoid them.

Although there are some possible health hazards that can occur for women seeking intermittent fasting as a healthy eating habit, this is only the exception to the rule. If you will follow the advice on how to prevent the side effects that we have discussed, you are more than likely to have a pleasant and beneficial experience as you begin this journey. Even ibuprofen has been known to cause everything from diarrhea to shortness of breath in some people, but I doubt that you consider these side effects every time you get a headache! Rest assured that with careful planning and self-awareness, intermittent fasting will help the large majority of women achieve their weight loss and fitness goals

Chapter 5: Why You Won't Binge on Intermittent Fasting

Understanding Binge Eating

It is in fact quite normal to overeat. In a society and culture filled with wonderfully delicious and delectable foods, it is not uncommon to indulge or overindulge at times. Having a wonderful entree or dessert and having a tough time restraining yourself from stopping when you know you are full is quite normal. But how do we differentiate this from binge eating? Where and how do you draw the line between simply overeating and binge eating?

As described, overeating may occur periodically when you are tempted with a favorite meal, delectable dessert, or even a special occasion where there is just too much food to choose from. While you still end up eating more than you should, these occurrences happen on an infrequent basis (normally with a large time span in between). Binge eating on the other hand is the complete opposite. Recurrent episodes of indulging without giving your body time to purge is a sure tell sign of binge eating. Often times you will also feel both emotional and physical distress (eating until the point of discomfort). When these experiences happen, it is important to understand and assess the cause to better diagnose what the real problem is.

Understanding Differences Between Overeating and Binge Eating

Since we know that overeating from time to time is normal, but binge eating is not, it can sometimes be extremely hard to understand the difference between the two, especially when beginning or practicing intermittent fasting. Here are a few associations with binge eating to help determine whether or not you are simply overeating or teetering on the edge of binging:

- Eating faster or much more rapidly than you normally do or should.

- Eating until you feel uncomfortably full. (This can sometimes be mistaken for a "full" feeling, but is much more intense. In some cases, it could even be painful.)

- Eating or consuming large amounts of food even when you don't feel physically hungry.

- Eating alone or by yourself because you feel embarrassed by how much food you are consuming. (You may also have a "disgusted" feeling with yourself.)

- Feeling depressed or guilty after eating or consuming food.

Binging, or eating far more than you should in one sitting, is the enemy of weight loss. Unfortunately, however, many people struggle against binge eating and fall prey to it. Especially those who have already been disappointed by a diet in the past. When this happens, it is important to keep in mind that past failure doesn't mean future failure when it comes to dieting, a person needs to discover their inspiration or motivation within them to sustain a fasting program that fits organically with their lifestyle.

Reasons for binge eating can be many and varied. It can have an emotional connection, such as depression or anxiety, or be a stress-related coping mechanism, or merely a habit developed over a long period of time, and one that can be very difficult to break. Once the root cause of binge eating is identified, it must be either dealt with to pave the road for breaking the habit of binge eating, or if the timing isn't right for whatever reason(s), then the cause and potential solution should be documented for use when a more appropriate time is desired.

For those who have struggled with overeating in the past, it can be a significant concern when deciding whether or not to practice intermittent fasting. The concern is that by fasting for an extended period, you will grow so hungry, you won't be able to stop yourself from binging once you break your fast. However,It should actually be looked at the other way because you have invested the time and effort to attain important goals in your life, so you can't destroy that progress by binge eating – finding something else to fill that void is key.

Binge Eating, Intermittent Fasting and Intuition

While no official studies have been published in this issue, many case studies can be used to help downplay this fear of overeating. These are important, as the ability to learn from people who went through what you are contemplating about undertaking or perhaps are experiencing right now can potentially help to save you valuable time and frustration down the road.

The most significant gift that intermittent fasting can give to the overeater is the chance to listen to their body. We hear this advice all the time, listen to your body, and it will tell you when to eat. For many who are overweight, and prone to overeating, we have lost that ability to listen to our bodies. We feel hungry all the time, or once we start eating, we stop looking to our stomachs. It's easy to get stuck in a rut and hard to get out of it, it might take a significant life event for a "wake up call" to take place and for change to happen – even if we lose the signal that enables us to listen to our bodies, sometimes life just slaps us in the face and shouts out WAKE UP, IT'S TIME FOR A CHANGE!

But something different starts to happen after a week or two of intermittent fasting. During your 16-hour fasts, you will get hungry, especially during the first weeks. You will feel hungry at breakfast time, but you can resist it. Then eventually something fascinating happens, a little after breakfast time, the hunger goes away. Even though you didn't eat breakfast, you don't feel hungry anymore!

You think that the hunger you were feeling is gone, and you have full control over when you can eat now so you go on with your morning, but in a few hours, the hunger comes back. It is stronger this time, but manageable. You wait until your lunch break, and then head out for lunch. This is the first moment of truth. Will your sandwich and salad satisfy you, or will you be driven to overeat? You may feel the urge to eat more to try and catch up on your food intake from what you "missed out on" at breakfast time, but discipline has to be taken to settle into this big lifestyle change.

What many people report, is being able to feel satisfied with less food than they were eating before? Why? Because you have learned to listen to your body, actually to feel the hunger, and so you can also feel when the craving has subsided. Plus as you eat less, your stomach will shrink down a bunch quicker than you think and as a result you will need less food to be happy and content like it was prior to your fasting.

Additional Triggers of Binge Eating:

When deciding to try intermittent fasting, there are definitely some key things to keep in mind to help avoid binge eating. Contrary to what you may believe, binge eating can actually be caused by other factors than just not eating for long periods of time. When you are just beginning or in the process of practicing intermittent fasting you can help both your body and your mind steer clear of binge eating by making sure you don't add insult to injury by triggering it without realizing. Here are a few ways you can trigger binge eating without even realizing you are doing it:

- Many individuals struggle with binge eating due to particular foods that actually trigger their binging episodes. As a rule of thumb, foods that are higher in carbohydrates and fats can cause the release of the hormone serotonin in the brain which can lead to a feeling of satisfaction and pleasure. For this reason, eating foods that you know you like or crave (sometimes referred to as comfort foods) can significantly increase the chances of triggering a binge eating episode. When trying to start or follow intermittent fasting, try and avoid these foods and replace them with something else - get creative, buy or prepare food or meals that you might not otherwise have.

- Eating out, especially at restaurants, can increase the risks for binge eating. Not only can eating out increase binge eating because of portion size - contrary to what you may believe, restaurants are notorious for larger than recommended portion sizes, but it can also trigger binge eating due to the overwhelming amount of food choices on the menu. If you pair these two factors with going to your favorite restaurant (think back to comfort food), you can easily end up ordering or eating too much. This doesn't mean that you can't do it, but just be aware of the increased risks and difficulties when you decide to go out for a meal.

- Depending upon your exercise patterns and regimes, eating patterns may follow suit as well. If you are someone who goes to the gym or likes to work out all the time, you are obviously burning a much higher number of calories per day than your friend sitting at home on the couch watching television. While this is great, be cautious of changes to your workout trends or programs, especially if the change is a decrease in the amount of time or work you were putting in before. Reducing the amount of time or effort you have been doing with your workouts may not immediately register with your body's routine and expectation for food replenishment. To avoid unwanted changes to your body's appearance, cutting down on the frequency of your workouts, or the amount of time you spend at the gym means reducing the number of calories you were eating as well. Since your body may not expect this right away, you may find yourself binge eating more than you should until your body has chance to catch up and understand its new lower energy requirement.

- Believe it or not, the nature of a family setting can affect binge eating. Often times, especially for children, the way in which they are taught to soothe themselves or cope with emotions has a direct correlation with food and eating. When beginning or practicing intermittent fasting be aware of this situation and its implications. As an adult, you may not even realize that as a child you already made an association with food as a soothing and coping method for various problems.

- Changes in your daily life or habits can also have an effect on binge eating. Depending upon the circumstances, things such as an increase in workload, stress, free time, and health habits (such as smoking) can influence your eating habits. Being mindful of these situations can help you identify whether you are eating more because you need to eat more or if you are eating more because you "think" you need to

- The factors that influence the development of binge eating can be complex. They can range from biological make up, to social conditions and your environment. When beginning or actively practicing intermittent fasting, be alert and conscious of certain events that you feel may bring on possible binge eating. While there are a plethora of different scenarios to be aware of, unfortunately there is no way to tell which may be the biggest influence on you. Also keep in mind I am not saying to give up your comfort foods all together, I certainly don't, but you will need to be aware of your personality type. If you are a person that really struggles to eat comfort foods in moderation then it is going to take a lot more discipline to keep on top of it than someone that is able keep those guilty pleasures to a minimum sticking to the 80/20 if possible..

Mindfulness, a Way to Avoid Binge Eating

Based more along the lines of psychology, mindfulness can help play a big role in preventing binge eating. While there is bound to be some initial skepticism in the beginning, those who stick with and incorporate these practices into their everyday lives (especially when practicing intermittent fasting) can expect to see helpful benefits in dealing with the urges to binge, especially when they occur sporadically. These practices have been shown to be effective and beneficial in helping a person overcome abnormal eating behaviors which can be a huge factor in triggering binge eating. But what are these practices and how do we apply them?

How Mindfulness Works

Before we begin talking about all the ways that mindfulness can help reduce binge eating, it is probably first more important to understand and recognize just what mindfulness is and what it means. Mindfulness is a mental state achieved by focusing on one's awareness and sensations in the present time ("being in the moment"). While in this state, you are able to calmly acknowledge and accept your own feelings, thoughts, and bodily sensations which allow you to use them as a therapeutic technique to relax and become even more aware of what is going on.

Generally speaking, mindfulness involves an awareness of what we are experiencing and going through moment by moment, second by second, frame by frame. This can include an awareness of what we are thinking, how we are feeling, and the understanding of the outside environment we are engaged with. Mindfulness doesn't end there however. Mindfulness is also the practice of *actually* accepting those thoughts and emotions that you are experiencing and using them to realize what is going on and why. By not passing judgement on the present moments going on around you, you can better listen, understand, and comprehend what your body is experiencing.

Benefits of Practicing Mindfulness

So what are some of the benefits of practicing mindfulness when doing intermittent fasting and striving to avoid binge eating? Well, here are some key ways in which being mindful can help prevent binge eating and boost your intermittent fasting dedication and practice.

Mindful Eating

By practicing mindful eating habits, a person can create and increase better awareness of thoughts, emotions, feelings, and behaviors related to what and why they are eating. While often at times eating disorders (especially binge eating) can affect and numb emotions, practicing mindfulness can help you personally reflect on why you are feeling this way, what triggers lead to it, and what you can do. Below are some useful mindfulness tips to help you along the way.

1. Make sure your body is in-tune with your brain.

Slowing down is one of the best, and maybe most direct, ways to get your body and mind to really establish a connection and communicate about nutrition. Since the body actually sends its satiation signal (which is the feeling of fullness which triggers the suppression of hunger) about 15-25 minutes after the brain, often times we end up unconsciously overeating. By slowing down, you can help give your body a chance to catch up to your brain and therefore adequately receive the signals to eat the right amount or simply stop eating.

Here are some relatively simple ways to slow down and get your body and mind in-tune while eating:

- o Take a load off, sit down to eat. Sitting down to eat can help signify that you actually have the time to accomplish what you are trying to do. Standing while eating or eating on the go can distract your mind (and body) from what is really going on - and more importantly, distract from when you are full.

- o Chewing your food slowly. Chewing your food slowly is another great, and relatively simple, way to get your body and mind on the same page. Chewing each bite for say 20-25 times not only slows down your eating since it is taking you longer, but also allows you to better enjoy your food as well.

- o If this still doesn't help, try setting down your utensils in between bites or making sure to take a drink of water (or whatever you are having to drink). Adding additional time between your food consumption gives the body and mind more time to get in sync.

o If all else fails, try making sure you engage in conversation, or if you are alone, find an object around you and describe, think, or talk about it. While this may seem counterproductive, since you are making your mind wander to something else, you are still limiting or slowing down your eating, thus allowing the body and mind better time to communicate.

2. Figure out your body's personal hunger signals

Is it emotion or needs?

Often times when it comes to doing something, we listen to our minds first, then our bodies second. By practicing mindfulness however, we may discover more wisdom and truth by reversing that order and turning to our bodies first. Rather than eating when we get the emotional signals sent from our mind (these can vary and be associated with many different reasons like stress, anger, loneliness, and even just plain old boredom), we can listen to what our bodies are telling us instead and adjust our course of action. Listening to when our bodies tell us something, rather than our mind, can help gauge the real reason behind why we are wanting food. Is it because our stomach is growling or our energy is low, or is it because we had a stressful day at work or are bored because there is nothing to do on a rainy afternoon? Genuine mindful eating is actually taking the time to listen to what your body is really saying and sometimes putting your mind on the back burner for a minute.

If you find yourself struggling to distinguish between the two, here are some questions you can ask yourself that may help you determine the real reason.

- o   What are my hunger signals?
- o   What types of situations spark my emotional hunger?
- o   What happened to me today that may influence the reasons why I feel this way?
- o   When was the last time I ate?
- o   What happened at home, work, school, etc, today?
- o   What kind of foods did I last eat?

3. Create and establish healthy eating environments.

Another great way to practice mindful eating is by not wondering around looking through the pantry and cabinets or deciding to eat at random places and times. Instead, try to think and connect proactively (rather than "reactively") about your meal times, foods and snacks. By doing this, you can help to create and develop healthy environment cues about what to eat, when to eat it and how much to eat. This will also help in wiring your brain in a way so that it can help you avoid developing associations with eating patterns and habits (i.e. getting the urge to eat every time you get on the bus or go for a drive in your car).

Creating and establishing a healthy eating environment can also be a huge help by limiting temptations and giving you access to "healthier amounts of healthy food". By putting food away and keeping it in designated places, it can help make you more aware of what you have, where it is, and if you really need it. Limiting your eating to designated places like the kitchen or dining room can also be a plus. Since you are more likely to mindlessly eat or overindulge when you are busy or multitasking, having a designated spot to eat allows you to connect with your food and not worry about anything else.

Finally, while you don't have to plan or strategize your food consumption down to each individual bite, it is important to understand and realize that you may have to adjust and change your eating habits throughout the year to accommodate different times and occasions. Planning ahead, and being mindful of the environment can help you better assess the situation, have a plan, and make sure you stick to it. By doing this, you are more likely to eat the amount your body needs in the moment rather than over indulging, or worse, under eating in the moment and then indulging more later.

4. Be aware of your motivations

While this can be a tricky and troublesome balance, ideally it is not impossible to find foods which are nourishing, satisfying, and comforting, all at the same time. Assuming that you are not a big fan of say spinach, think back to that first time you ate it. How appealing was it before you tried it? How about after? If you found that after eating the spinach you actually liked it, then that goes to show that when we slow down and eat healthy foods (like spinach) we often end up enjoying them more than what we may have originally anticipated we would. As we practice mindfulness and begin eating a healthier and a greater variety of foods, we are also less inclined to feel the urge to binge on foods that we have already labeled as "comfort" foods. This will ultimately allow you to find a greater variety of foods both mentally and physically satisfying - as opposed to just a few.

5. Gain an in-depth connection with your food.

Unless you are a hunter or a farmer, in recent times, we have all become increasingly disconnected from the actual food we eat. In today's day and age no one ever worries about where a meal comes from (except for maybe the grocery store packaging). While you may find yourself saying, "why does this even matter?", the truth of it is that eating actually offers us an incredible opportunity to connect more with the world around us, its elements, and even to each other.

Pausing to consider everything that has gone into a meal (from those who prepared it, to those who filled the shelves, transported it, and even those who planted, harvested, or procured the raw ingredients) it's hard not to be amazed and grateful at the same time. Taking time to consider these things can not only help you better connect with the food you are eating, but also give you a deeper appreciation for things like tradition, recipes, or the places that it has come from.

When you consider everything that has gone into the meal you are eating, it becomes second nature to experience and express appreciation for all of the things that have gone into allowing you this opportunity to eat. Considering things like this will also help give you more mindfulness about all the steps, processes, factors, and other things that make up the meal in front of you. When we do this, it can give us a better perspective about the world around us and can even lead to wiser choices about sustainability and health in our food.

6. Pay attention to your plate

Distracted eating, which can be caused by multitasking while eating, is a recipe for disaster. Not listening to our body's needs and wants can lead to choices that are counteractive and counterproductive. When we get distracted, it becomes harder and harder to listen to what our body is telling us about what it needs and the foods it wants. Simple or "single-task" eating, which is exactly what it sounds like - just eating, is a great way to connect the food in front of you with what your body wants and needs. Try eating your meals without any screens or distractions and enjoying the company and conversation of those you are sharing it with.

By understanding and practicing mindfulness when we eat, we can gain a better perspective on a wide variety of factors that can help prevent binge eating. By doing so, we can develop a connection between the food we eat and what our minds and bodies really need. The reality is we do live, work, and eat in the real world, and the real world is a busy place. Taking our perspectives from our formal practices of slowing down, listening to our bodies, creating small practices and rituals, and even considering all the factors that went into our meal on a regular basis brings not only more mindfulness into our daily meals, but gives us a better connection to fuel our bodies in the right way.

Additional benefits of practicing mindfulness:

- Helping to eliminate Stress and Anxiety

Often times binge eating is a result of using food to cope with increased stress and anxiety from outside (or even inside) sources. Using mindfulness can be helpful and therapeutic in effectively learning how to deal with certain "stressors" that may in fact trigger binge eating. By processing your emotions, rather than hiding behind them, not only can you determine the problem, but you can also help eliminate it.

- Making Peace with Your Body and Food

Learning to accept your body in the present moment can be a tremendous help and benefit in suppressing binge eating and coming to terms with your feelings and the food you eat. By not casting judgement on yourself, you can gain a greater acceptance of the present moment, emotions, and food, thus leading to better overall feelings and approval.

Intermittent Fasting and Willpower

The truth is complicated. Intermittent fasting will take some amount of willpower in the beginning. You will have to work hard to skip breakfast or endure one 24 hour fast. But over time, your willpower will get stronger. Willpower is like a muscle, we only have a limited amount of willpower strength, but we can gain more through practice. It may take some experimentation to figure out the ideal fasting schedule that works with how you live your life on a daily basis, but when something clicks, it will have you thinking that anything is possible and you will find your world on a refreshed and an exciting new trajectory.

Consider your journey into intermittent fasting like an exercise for your willpower and your intuition. Although it will be a challenge at first, through this lifestyle, you will increase your overall willpower, and learn how to listen to your body. When your body speaks and you listen and respond in perfect harmony, it feels like a well-oiled machine that can be seen externally and perhaps even more importantly - felt internally as well.

This increase in overall willpower can lead to many positive changes in the rest of your life. Increased willpower in eating can also lead to increased willpower towards exercise. Do you have a hard time finding the motivation and energy to go to the gym or stick to a workout plan? With intermittent fasting, you'll have boosted power, and increased willpower. Just think of the possibilities, it can lead to new ways of thinking about how you interact with the world and bring on a new realization of a more confident version of yourself!

Now is the time to remind yourself that significant

changes take time. Intermittent fasting is not a quick fix! Yes, if you follow the plan, you will see results within the first few weeks. However, if you want real lasting change, to your weight, your health, and your lifestyle, you will need to be patient. Promise to give intermittent fasting at least two or three months, and then you can check back in to see just how far you've come. In order to see how you have truly benefited from intermittent fasting, it is important to keep track of the tangible metrics daily that matter most to you such as your weight change, clothing sizing, lifestyle and even the dollar amount saved as less food will be run through your local grocery stores checkout counters.

Chapter 6: Popular Ways to Fast Intermittently

To be successful, consistent, and regular while fasting intermittently, you need to find a method that can fit into your lifestyle, one thing you do need to realize is that if you eat more calories than you burn then it doesn't matter which weight loss method you use you will fail. Weight loss can be purely hormonal in some cases but with the majority of people it is a numbers game. The weight loss equation I use it as follows:

Take your body weight and convert it into pounds then multiply that number by 13, this gives you your rough maintenance level of calories you can consume to maintain your current body weight. If you want to lose weight then you obviously need to eat less than that number. A good amount to subtract from that maintenance number is 500 calories. You don't want to cut too much out as it will make it harder to sustain and also drain you of your energy.

These number of course are just a guide as there is no real way of knowing what your exact maintenance level of calories are as that is a very individual thing that depends on so many different factors. You may have to play around with the numbers slightly depending on your activity level and lifestyle but I would advise you to start with that number and run with it for a few weeks and then adjust it from there. For the most part I have had success with this equation so I know it works.

If you have concerns about what number is best for you and your body, then you can speak with your trusted healthcare professional. Having the knowledge of your medical history, they will be able to guide you to a healthy number of calories for you individually.

Another thing you might like to do at the start is track your calories. Calories can build up very quickly without even realizing it. I would strongly suggest tracking your macros at least for the first few weeks. You will find that over a 2-3 week period you would have probably eaten most of the foods that you eat regularly and from there you will be better placed to eye ball your food servings rather than measuring and tracking everything that goes into your mouth.

There are plenty of free apps you can download to make tracking incredibly easy. I like to use the app "my fitness pal" it makes tracking macros effortless and barely takes any time at all to implement. The free version is fine so there is no need to upgrade to the paid version. A side note is to only use it to calculate your calories, don't pay any attention to the caloric number they tell you to eat as I have found that it under estimates what you can eat and makes it less sustainable.

Once you start to see your results going in the right direction, you will understand exactly what needs to be followed from a calorie intake and exercise stand point. It then comes down to simply sticking with the plan and being consistent until you reach the goals you set for yourself. Half the battle is getting into a good routine that works for you personally so you can build momentum and tick off those small goals along the way. This builds an inner confidence which will carry you through to your end goal.

Here are six popular ways to go about intermittent fasting

1. 16/8 Method:

This method is by far the most popular and probably the most sustainable in my opinion. It consists of not eating for 16 hours each day and then having an 8-hour window to consume all of your calories. You can split those calories up within that 8 hour feeding window however your wish. I normally have 2 to 3 meals. During the fasting period, it is okay to drink water or beverages that have zero calories like tea or straight black coffee with no fillers. Generally, you avoid eating anything after dinner and by the time lunch rolls around the next day, it will probably have been around 16 hours in between meals. If you are someone that naturally skips breakfast, you may find it easy to adopt this method, also known as the "Lean-gains protocol."

Many health experts recommend that women change the regime slightly and eat after 14-15 hours because they tend to do better with a somewhat shorter fast. For this to be an effective weight loss method, it is essential that you eat a good amount of healthy meals during your 8-hour non-fasting window along with a couple guilty pleasures, if you are able to have them in moderation of course, rather than filling it with a bunch of processed or refined foods. Many people find it easy to adjust to this method of intermittent fasting, and it becomes effortless to them. Pros of this method are, it saves you money because you are eating fewer meals; it burns fat and you do not have to count calories as it can become quite difficult to over eat since your eating all of your calories in such a short window, however as I mentioned earlier I do recommend you count calories for the first few weeks. This version of fasting can be used by your average person looking to drop a few pounds as well as people who consider themselves gym addicts all the way through to endurance athletes. This method was developed Martin Berkhan.

2. Eat-Stop-Eat:

To pull this off, you do a complete 24-hour fast either

once or twice a week. The best way to accomplish this is to go from the end of a meal to the same meal-time the following day. An example is if you finish dinner at 7pm on a Saturday, you will not eat again until 7pm on Sunday or whenever you eat dinner. You can also go from breakfast to breakfast or from lunch to lunch, whatever is more convenient for your lifestyle. Picking the same day or days each week to implement this fasting approach is recommended. Remember, we are creatures of habit and our bodies will adjust to our new lifestyle once they recognize a regular pattern developing.

Again, water and any other non-caloric beverages are excellent, and as always aim for healthy foods over junk. You may find it too hard to go 24 hours right away and need to build that up over time, you can always begin with a 12-14 hour fast then build up to the 16/8 method and then eventually to the eat stop eat regime. This method takes a lot of self-discipline and isn't my preferred option, but it may be preferable for you. You could always follow a normal eating pattern most of the week and focus on this type of fasting for just a day or two. One of the biggest pros of this method is that it requires less willpower because you know that your fast is only a couple days per week. You can also somewhat eat what you want as long as it is in moderation. The first week or two may be a bit of a shock to the body with a full day or two of fasting per week, but over time, the mind and body can align and work together after understanding the beneficial reasons as to why this change in eating behavior is occurring. Brad Pilon is credited with creating this method of intermittent fasting.

3. The 5:2 Method/Diet:

This method is very similar to Eat-Stop-Eat but does not require you to fast for a full 24 hours. To do this technique, you would usually eat normally five days a week and restrict yourself to 500-600 calories per day twice a week. Some studies suggest women are supposed to aim for 500 calories and men for 600. This is usually broken up into two small meals for the day. The two low-calorie counting days in which you somewhat fast should not be consecutive. This method has had the least amount of research done, and critics are quick to point out that no scientific studies are showing its effectiveness. Therefore I cannot recommend it nor do I personally know anybody who has done it. This method does require you to keep track of the calories you are eating, so that's also a disadvantage. However, the proof is in the pudding, so if you decide to move forward with this fasting methodology and get the results that you are after and see it being sustainable long-term, then keep up the good work!

4. The Warrior Method/Diet:

Fast all day, and then feast at night if you want to try this. This reminds me, and perhaps you too, of the Viking movies where the warriors come back to the lodge, and there are crates and plates of abundant foods awaiting. During the day, you are allowed to snack on vegetables as long as they are raw. Then, at night you eat one giant meal. You technically get a 4-hour window to eat at night, but most users of this method stick to one large meal. This way of fasting/dieting agrees with the "Paleo" diet in which people try to stick to healthy, natural, unprocessed foods that resemble what foods are found in Nature. Of all the menus to become popular in recent years, the warrior diet was the first to involve a type of intermittent fasting. Pros of this method are first of all, you can eat appropriate snacks, and secondly it is very, very healthy. The con is that you have to monitor yourself really closely and make sure you are going with healthy food choices. Other than raw veggies, you are fasting for a full 20 hours every day. If you tend to have a very busy lifestyle during the day and don't really think about food too much or get very hungry for anything other than a good, hearty dinner, then this version might be worth a try. This method is credited to Ori Hofmekler. There are some similarities to the Ramadan or the 30 day Muslim fast, with Ramadan, of course, being mostly spiritually motivated.

5. Alternate Day Fasting:

If you are up to the challenge, you can try to fast every other day. This is an extreme method that should not be attempted by beginners, but you can choose to go with a full-on fast or to limit your calorie intake to about 500 every other day. Many of the scientific studies that showed the health benefits of intermittent fasting used a sort of alternate day fasting. Ideally, while using this method, you are still eating at least once a day, with your fast going from dinnertime to dinnertime every other day. The pros of this type of fasting are, you will experience rapid weight loss-with people averaging a 1 to 2 pound drop per week, It requires less willpower as you can eat a little on fasting days and then look forward to eating more the next day. The con is that you have to be very, very careful to not binge on your eating days. If you have tried this approach before and gave it at least a few weeks for your body to adjust, and it still wasn't working for you and your lifestyle, then try another fasting method that isn't so demanding – you may not get significant results nearly as quickly, but you are after something that is sustainable for months and maybe even years depending on how your goals change and evolve as you age. Dr. James Johnson created this type of intermittent fasting when he realized it is apparently impossible for most working people to maintain a consistent calorie restriction by pure willpower.

6. Meal Skipping:

You do not need to follow an incredibly strict schedule to get some benefits from intermittent fasting. Today's market-oriented forces have convinced the majority of people that we need to eat every few hours, or we will start losing muscle mass and begin to starve. If you are not feeling hungry or are too busy to stop and eat, then only skip that certain meal that you would normally eat during that particular part of the day. This actually has some benefits. Generally speaking, and discomfort aside, the human body is configured in advance to handle famine, so skipping a meal or two will not cause you any damage. Skipping a meal or two when it works out best for you is a spontaneous intermittent fast done in a very natural way. Just make sure that when you are eating, it is healthy food. Skipping meals at times just happens by accident where maybe you have a busy morning that wasn't planned, and before you know it, it's lunchtime and your stomach didn't even miss its normal intake of cereal, a bagel, or a smoothie. Whether intentional or accidental, skipping a meal here and there can help with weight loss and help you reach other important goals that you may have. The good aspect about this method is that it's easy to do whenever you are up for it, and you can notice and feel incremental results along the way.

These are just a few of the popular versions of

intermittent fasting, there are many more out there that you can do your own research on and follow, or alternately you can make your own plan that suits you.

My Personal Method

I myself don't place to many rules on how I implement fasting into my life. I aim to fast for the first 4-6 hours upon waking up. I will then eat 1 or 2 pieces of fruit to fill a gap if I need to. I will then have a small meal a couple of hours later that is mainly protein, fat and vegetable based before consuming most of my calories with big meals at night as I find this to be the most enjoyable and sustainable way for me to follow intermittent fasting. Eating right before bed is not a problem as long as you get a good 6-8 hours of fasting during sleep followed by the 4-6 hours when you wake.

Another thing to note is I don't let my intermittent fasting lifestyle prevent me from partaking in breakfast events and get togethers with family and friends. Sometimes I might have a family breakfast outing I have been invited to, if that is the case then I don't fast on those days. These obviously don't come up all that often but when they do I break the rules and enjoy breakfast, life is too short and it's about living and having fun so don't deprive yourself from going to the odd occasion, go and enjoy yourself without feeling guilty about not following your eating pattern on that particular day, just get back on track the next day as per normal. One day of going against your new lifestyle is not going to effect your long term results.

No matter which approach of intermittent fasting you decide to start with and try out, there are going to be times where you just want to go back to how things were because it was easier that way. The healthiest and happiest version of yourself won't come from eating whatever and whenever you want – this was maybe the case when you were a kid and your metabolism was running fast, but as we age, our metabolism slows down and we have to adjust our food intake and calorie count accordingly to maintain the same ratio between our height to weight.

You don't have to do any of this fasting stuff alone either, reach out to those that you trust and love the most for much-needed support along the way, the support of your loved ones and encouragement is going to make your journey so much easier rather than having it become a tough slog that ends up making you more unhappy than you were before you started. An excellent scenario would be that both you and your spouse want to do fasting, and you can do it together to motivate each other. When one of you is losing focus and getting off track, the other is there to steer them back and vice versa, this is also a great way to approach your exercise routine. Fasting and exercising in collaboration with someone you love has many positive elements including building a stronger relationship and bond, and who isn't open to an amazing beneficial byproduct like this from happening?

Chapter 7: Exercise and Intermittent Fasting

One common question that people have when doing intermittent fasting is whether or not it is safe and healthy to exercise either aerobically or anaerobically while they are, say, "running on empty." But, if done correctly, the combination can help you burn lots of your body's fat reserves quickly. Additionally, maintaining a regular exercise routine is vital for your mental and physical health and well being. So, in fact, exercising in a fasted state is a great way to become fat adapted and improve your mental health at the same time.

You've already heard the adage, 80% diet, 20% exercise to combine dieting with training. This is true! Imagine if we could make our body burn more fat for fuel while at rest, as well as have it burn fat more efficiently during exercise. Like I mentioned in a previous chapter most of us have 40,000 calories of fat in our bodies at any given time and around 1,200 calories of muscle glycogen or sugar. Imagine how far or how much we could exercise if we had access to that 40,000-calorie fuel tank. That's 33 times the amount of energy fuel! So, perhaps next time you run out of energy in the middle of an exercise routine, you will wish your body was in fat-burning mode instead of calorie-burning mode.

The first step to burning more fat during exercise is to make sure that you have what's called an "aerobic base." The way to build this base is thru aerobic heart rate training, which will raise what is known as your "aerobic capacity." Aerobic capacity is defined as the maximal amount of oxygen in milliliters (ml) that an athlete utilizes in one minute, per kilogram of body weight. In layman's terms, the higher the "aerobic base" or "capacity," the higher the body of work you can do in one minute. The best method I have found for heart rate training is Phil Maffetone's "MAF" training. If you would like to learn more about his method, then I would encourage you to google Phil Maffetone training.

What does this mean for exercise? Technically, by having a higher aerobic base, we boost the size and strength of our heart, the concentration of hemoglobin in our blood, the density of our capillaries, and the number of mitochondria in our muscles. The benefits expand beyond the scope of this book, but mostly by developing an aerobic base, we become healthier inside and out.

What this means for intermittent fasting is that when you are training in a fasted state, your body becomes superbly efficient at burning fat for fuel. From an aerobic aspect your body can more efficiently utilize oxygen and this, in turn, makes you more productive at exercise aerobically or anaerobically. You must first develop your aerobic base to enhance anaerobic exercise. You can check out Phil Maffetone's website for more details.

If you are looking to add muscle, fasting can help by increasing the production of certain hormones in your body. Other than weight training and getting the proper amount of sleep regularly, fasting has proven to be one of the most effective methods of increasing human growth hormone, or "HGH." Studies have also suggested that fasting in combination with regular exercise can increase the levels of testosterone in men and women. It's important for woman not to be scared by what I just mentioned with your testosterone levels increasing as this is just another hormone that can decrease your body fat and increase lean muscle and tone. Here are my recommendations for adding muscle:

- Don't push yourself too hard. If you are doing "cardio" exercise, as a test, make sure you can carry on somewhat of a conversation at the same time; otherwise, you may be pushing yourself too hard. When you are doing cardio exercise slowly, but for a long time is when your body is becoming more "fat adapted." That's when it is going into a ketogenic state. Always listen to your body, and stop if you start to feel dizzy or lightheaded.

- The 16/8 method, in particular, recommends scheduling your meals for when you plan to finish doing any moderate-to-intense exercise. Plan your high-intensity workouts for a time when you are getting ready to break your fast so that you can eat soon after your workout. Adequately scheduled, if your workout is very intense, you can follow it with a carbohydrate-rich snack which is a great time to consume your carbs as your body is like a sponge at that point and will soak up those calories with very little of them spilling over as fat.

- If you are lifting weights, make sure you are getting adequate protein or supplementing with adequate BCAAs. "Feast" on meals that are high in protein. Eating protein on a regular basis is vital to muscle growth and muscle retention. Protein is also very satiating.

- When planning your meals with workouts in mind, try combining fast-acting simple carbohydrates with a protein that will serve to stabilize your blood sugar after your workout. A banana and some peanut butter is a good example. You can also have a little fun with this post workout meal as simple sugars are best taken in at this time rather than you low GI types.

Here are some sample routines for nourishment while exercising when using intermittent fasting: Early Morning Exercise:

- Exercise fasted in the early morning: aerobic or anaerobic. Examples: a brisk walk on an incline and/or weights
- Take BCAAs before and after your training.
- Around Noon: Eat lunch. Aim for about 20-25% of your daily calorie intake.
- Around 3 PM: Snack on high-fat foods, nuts, and seeds.
- Between 4-5 PM: Eat dinner. This should be your most substantial meal of the day.
- Maybe have another light snack at around 7.30pm-8pm
- Fast from 8pm until noon the next day.
- Lunch Time Exercise: Take in some BCAAs before and after your workout
- Exercise fasted at lunch: aerobic or anaerobic. Again as examples: a brisk walk on an incline, or weights, if you did aerobic training the previous day then maybe do a weight training session on this day so you get the benefits of both.
- After exercising around 1-2pm: Eat lunch. Aim for 20-25% of your daily calorie intake.
- Around 3-4 PM: Snack on high-fat foods, nuts, and seeds

- Around 6 PM: Eat dinner. This meal's calories should approximate your lunches.
- Around 8-9 PM: Eat a light snack if needed.
- Fast from 9 pm or 10 pm until 1-2pm the next day.

You will likely not be working out every single day. So, on rest days, your biggest meal of the day should ideally be your first one instead of you're last but that's not written in stone as I like to switch these around. On rest days, you could aim to consume roughly 35-40% of your calories in your first meal, and eat a lot of protein and fat as part of this meal.

Is Exercise During Intermittent Fasting Okay?

You understand the meaning of intermittent fasting, but do not really know if it's alright to exercise during Intermittent fasting. Exercise during intermittent fasting is okay for the large majority of people. Engaging in mild and light bodyweight exercises is highly recommended. Ensure you stay hydrated and stop the exercise whenever you feel unable to cope with the exercise. There are some people however who even though feel great with a fasting lifestyle still struggle to keep the intensity up during exercise without any food in their body. They feel faint, dizzy and lethargic, if you are one of these people maybe schedule your workout a couple hours after you break your fast. Give your body time to digest your meal as you don't most of your energy going towards digestion during your workout when you need it to be put towards a great workout.

Intermittent fasting and your improvement of health

Fasting intermittently improves your health in the three primary ways discussed below.

Helps in developing healthy cells

When practicing intermittent fasting, your body cells undergo duress while enhancing their tendency to cope with stress. Through adapting and responding to the stress, it develops the ability to resist disease. Also, cells in a state of fasting will develop a self-eating process called autophagy (a natural process whereby the body breaks down and absorbs its cells and tissues). It involves the removal of waste for the cell and has been confirmed to help in the removal of non-functional proteins that are built up in the cell walls.

Helps in body Fat Loss

Your body usually stores fat for energy when you are fasting intermittently. Availability of carbohydrates (glucose) is limited when you do not eat for close to eight hours and above which makes the body facilitate the creation of energy through the process of burning fat.

Helps in Weight Loss

There's a considerable likelihood of reducing your appetite through intermittent fasting, which leads to consuming a lower amount of calories.

Can I exercise during the mornings of my intermittent fasting?

Most times, when you're fasting intermittently, the mornings are always a great time for exercise. This is because of the advantages accrued to exercising in the morning while fasting. Keep your workouts minimal and do not spend more than 1 hour exercising in this state. If you are training properly then you shouldn't be able to go beyond an hour anyway.

Exercises to try out when fasting include a mix or one of the following: cycling, brisk walking, bodyweight weight training, light jogging, weight training, yoga, swimming, hiking or a weights circuit.

Is exercise during Intermittent Fasting strenuous?

While starting intermittent fasting, you could have a hard time getting past the feeling of hunger when you wake in the morning even when you're not exercising! It's a great idea to find something to distract you from this feeling through exercises you love and enjoy. When you do this, you will easily feel a connection between your mind and body because you find it interesting.

Other forms of exercise you could try during intermittent fasting.

1. Dance/Zumba

Dancing helps you do away with your hunger state if it's something you enjoy doing. Several forms of dancing like the ballet dance, Zumba or dancing to hip-hop music are some variations.

2. A pump class

A pump class can be a great way to get some resistance training in for those people that dislike hitting the weights area of the gym on their own. It hits the entire body, it's social, you have an instructor making sure your technique is on point and with the smaller rest times in between exercises you will also get a cardio benefit out of it.

3. Tennis

Tennis is not only for the professionals, it's also useful for those doing intermittent fasting. It's usually preferred earlier in the day before the afternoon sun and it's also social.

4. Yoga

I mentioned this earlier but would like to elaborate on it, many Yoga Practitioners engage in yoga while on an empty stomach as it gives them a feeling of lightness that lets them focus purely on the bodily moves and breathing. The time you spend on Yoga as your form of workout in fasting mode depends on how much time you have.

5. Light Jogging

As mentioned earlier jogging is another activity you can do although I just wanted to elaborate quickly on this. Keeping in mind what I said earlier, you want to make sure you keep your heart rate at a point where you can still have somewhat of a conversation. With that in mind make sure you jog doesn't turn into a run and keep it short and sweet, 20 to 30 minutes at a steady rate while listening to your favorite podcast is ample.

Besides what I have mentioned, there are many many other activities that you can try which will keep your mind of eating during your fasted period as well as burning a few extra caries along the way. If you're a parent like me maybe get outside and kick a ball around with your kids or run around with them at the playground. This is a great one as not only will you burn calories but you get to see the enjoyment on their faces, create a tighter bond and create memories. I can tell you from my experience they are harder to keep up with and will push you harder than most personal trainers, or at least mine do.

Just remember, don't overdo things, always ensure to keep hydrated and whenever you notice any sign of weakness or dizziness you should stop instantly!. Exercises to avoid while doing intermittent fasting include: Crossfit, boxing and powerlifting since they are of a much higher intensity level.

Can Weight Training Help You Preserve Your Muscle During Intermittent Fasting?

Studies show that muscle loss can be prevented through weight loss as a result of intermittent fasting. The research was specifically carried out using 34 experienced weight trainers. They were divided into a group of two; the first group were placed on a restricted diet (expending their entire calories within 8 hours daily), and the other group followed a normal diet.

Each of these groups were given the same amount of protein and calories every day but weren't served the meals at the same time. At the end of the study, it was discovered that none of the groups had a weight or strength loss while only one group, the restricted group, had fat loss. The normal diet group did not lose any fat while the restricted group lost 1.6 kg of fat which is 3.5 pounds.

This is evidence of the fact that engaging in weight training three times a week while intermittent fasting can help preserve your muscle as a result of fat loss.

Studies on alternate-day fasting have also proven that 25-40 minutes bike riding twice a week can help during weight loss, to preserve your lean mass. Therefore, engaging in exercises during intermittent fasting is highly beneficial for you if you're looking forward to keeping your muscle.

Role of a Diet in Weight Loss

These are some things you can do to gain as much muscle as possible when you decide to use fasting as a means of losing weight. Weight training is one of the many exercises that can help you lose weight gradually and help maintain your muscle.

As earlier stated, research has proven that you have a high probability of losing some lean muscle when you lose weight as quickly as possible with intermittent fasting. What this means is that, when intermittent fasting, try not to reduce the intake of calories in one hit. Don't rush it. Stick to a particular amount of calories you think is best for you per day, week or month. Most experts suggest that a loss of 0.45 to 0.9 kilograms every week is healthy.

However, since the specific rate of weight loss varies from person to person, you may decide to go for the higher or lower end of this range. Another factor that plays a huge role in maintaining your muscle while fasting is the composition of your diet. During fasting, your body will not have the advantage of taking in the necessary nutrients you need, which is why protein intake should be taken seriously.

Protein is essential in your diet if you genuinely want to lose fat, so try to consume enough protein based foods. It has been discovered through different research that enough protein intake will help keep your muscle mass during the fat loss stage of your transformation.

IF is a widely used dietary plan where someone needs to fast longer than they do in overnight fasting. A classic example of IF is religious fasting. Other forms of Intermittent fasting include periodic fasting, time-restricted dieting, alternate-day fasting, and 5:2 diets.

IF probably doesn't lead to any more of a loss of muscle than other diets out there. However, including exercise particularly weight training to your IF regimen can aid in retaining your muscle that muscle which is so hard to earn but so easy to lose.

The decision to exercise while fasting is an individual thing. In some cases, fasting might not be as beneficial as you think, and it could affect your ideal exercise performance if you're a competitive athlete. Therefore, you should aim to lose weight slowly while taking in lots of protein to help keep your muscle mass in good shape while undergoing intermittent fasting.

Important Dietary Supplements That Helps Maintain Your Muscle

To preserve your muscle during intermittent fasting, there are dietary supplements you should consider taking at the appropriate time without it interfering with your weight loss results.

There are two supplements you should put to good use at this very crucial time. They are;

1. Creatine supplements

2. Protein supplements

Creatine supplements

Creatine is a natural molecule that occurs in your body, but it can be improved through the use of dietary supplements. Creatine supplements help support your muscles and are very useful in the improvement of your strength.

Protein supplements

Getting enough protein in through food alone can be tough, especially during a restricted eating window. Steak, chicken, eggs and other high protein food types are filling and eating enough of it can be a challenge and in many cases a chore. By using protein supplements, you'll be able to quickly get enough protein quicker and easier than having to eat those specific kinds of foods. Another thing to understand is after a workout you want to get protein to your muscles as quickly as possible, around 20 minutes from the time it goes into your mouth until the time it hits your muscle. The quickest way to get any nutrients to your muscles is to take it in liquid form. If you were to sit down and have an actual meal after you workout by the time you cut it, chew it, swallow it and digest it you have already missed that precious 20 minutes window where your muscles are crying out for replenishment. Protein supplements are a great way of improving your performances during exercise as well as recovery afterwards.

A few other supplements I include in my diet plan is fish oil which is essential for brain function. A lot of people struggle to get in enough omega 3 from food so in most cases I always recommend some type of omega 3 supplement.

Another one is magnesium, great in improving sleep quality and in turn aiding muscle recovery.

Supplements during Your Fasting Periods

The two supplements I have just spoke about are not necessary during shorter forms of intermittent fasting except when you're looking at gaining lean muscle, which everybody should be trying do to in my opinion. These supplements, when taken during your eating periods of intermittent fasting will help improve your lean muscle mass and overall strength. As long as you consume protein-rich meals during your feeding window, 16 hours of starvation shouldn't have adverse effects on your muscle.

So long as you aim to reduce your weight gradually, you have high chances of maintaining your muscle mass during intermittent fasting, especially. The area where people go wrong is they want to achieve their weight loss as fast as possible and their lack of patience leads to them severely under eating. This might have an immediate impact on the scale which you enjoy but it is a short term fix and will have you almost certainly losing muscle and having your weight loss come to a complete stop pretty quickly. Going down this road is what causes your metabolism to crash and makes any type of diet plan almost impossible to stick to long term. It's unhealthy and unnecessary.

Chapter 8: Tips and Tricks for Success

While each type of intermittent fasting is beneficial in its way, they can also each be very complicated and confusing to stick within both the long and the short term if you don't tackle them with the right mindset. The suggestions found in the following pages can make the process more comfortable, so it is recommended that you give them a try before throwing in the towel and going back to your old unhealthy or lazy eating habits.

Stay true to yourself:
While intermittent fasting can indeed provide you with a variety of healthy lifestyle changes, it doesn't mean it is going to be the right choice for everyone. While you should be able to make it through some fasts without slipping, once you have done so you are going to want to consider how difficult that period was for you. You will also need to think what your natural habits are like when it comes to eating and what your overall relationship with food is like in general. It is essential to keep in mind that intermittent fasting is not so much a diet as it is a lifestyle, which means you should focus on long-term sustainability and not think about it as a short-term solution like you would with many actual diets.

This long-term commitment is why you are going to want to seriously ask yourself if you are going to be able to commit to fasting regularly in the long term, if not with the first type of intermittent fasting then you can possibly try a second or third type. If you have a long way to go when it comes to meeting your weight loss goals, then you may want to start with something milder than intermittent fasting and instead work up to it once you have gotten into the habit of eating healthy first. Starting off with a style of eating that has an extreme learning curve can lead to early failure that can affect you mentally and make you less likely to try again. Remember the best method of weight loss is the most sustainable method of weight loss for you personally and that method will differ from person to person. Intermittent fasting is great but by no means is it the only way.

Be aware of what your body is trying to tell you:
While adjusting to intermittent fasting will almost always come with some side effects, it is important to remember that these are supposed to fade with time which means you are going to want to remain in touch with your body to ensure you don't end up hurting yourself in the process. If you find yourself experiencing more prolonged or more severe symptoms, it is essential to stop immediately instead of powering through. Maintaining your overall health is critical when it comes to maximizing the results from intermittent fasting, and you can't do that if your body is reacting

negatively to the process. Remember we are doing this to improve our body and health not make it worse so listen to the things your body is telling you and never try to push yourself past your limits, if you do, you could find yourself passing out from hunger, or possibly worse.

Don't expect too much, too soon:
It is essential to keep in mind that initially, when you switch to an intermittent fasting plan you may in some cases not lose weight for the first week or so as your body reacts to the change. From there, you are likely to experience a period where you enjoy larger than average amounts of weight loss for a period of time. This will not last however, and as your body fully adapts to the change, you will likely start to see weight loss of about 1 pound per week, which is the average amount of healthy weight loss recommended by experts.

Additionally, you are going to need to keep in mind that everyone hits weight loss plateaus, regardless of how strict they are being with their chosen weight loss plan. This is an unavoidable part of losing weight and if you take that as an excuse to mix things up with a new type of intermittent fasting or to naturally fall off the wagon you are going to be doing yourself a great disservice. Changing horses midstream is only going to confuse your body without making you lose weight any faster and falling off the wagon has never done anyone any good regardless of the specifics of the situation. Only change your method of fasting if the one you are currently following is not working with your lifestyle not because your weight loss has slowed down. Stay the course, and you will be back on track before you know it.

Don't let yourself make excuses:
While it is essential not to get started on a new intermittent fasting plan when your schedule is hectic, or you have extra stress or anxiety on your plate, it is also important to make sure you don't keep putting it off every time something new comes up. Life is always going to be busy, that is why one of the benefits of intermittent fasting is having more time each fasting day. At some point, the reasons you have for putting it off are merely going to be excuses to avoid getting started. Be frank with yourself and understand that there is always going to be something standing in your way from making positive life changes. You just need to power through it if you ever hope to see real success. The perfect time doesn't exist so stop waiting for it. A saying I really like that gets this message across is "life isn't about waiting for the storm to pass, it's about learning how to dance in the rain"

At some point, all you can do is say enough is enough and get down to business. After all, the only person that can motivate you to stick with a healthy intermittent fasting diet plan in the long term is you. This is why it is so important not to let yourself down. If you truly commit to finding personal success when it comes to your weight loss goals, then there should be nothing that can stop you. It is as simple as that.

Set the right goals:

Once you do start your preferred intermittent fasting plan, you are going to want to take into account that a 3,500-calorie deficit is going to lead to the loss of one pound of fat. Keep in mind that this equation doesn't take muscle growth into the equation. This means that if you are exercising regularly, then you may end up losing less weight per week on the scale, but still end up looking and feeling better regardless. If you find yourself feeling discouraged based on the results from the scale, it is essential to consider how long it took you to reach your current weight and fitness level and then give yourself a comparable period to get back to where you need to be. Getting to your current point didn't happen overnight, and there is no reason to expect that changing things up drastically will lead to overnight results either. Learn to enjoy the process and let the results be a by-product of that.

Start off the right way:

If you have never gone without a meal for 12 hours in your life, then you are likely going to find the best results by starting with an intermittent fasting plan that limits when you eat to 12 hours a day and work your way up from there. It is essential to take things slow and steady and not to push yourself too fast too soon as you will likely experience side effects by doing so. Jumping right into a more severe type of intermittent fasting can lead to failure which can make it difficult to give the process the fair shot it deserves.

If even 12 hours seems like a stretch, there is no reason you can't start with an even more manageable timeframe and then work up from there. When you start intermittent fasting, you are not being judged based on how other people have found success. It is more about finding success for yourself and sticking to it in the long run, than meeting any specific goal, especially right out of the gate. Whatever you decide, it is essential to try and stick with it as diligently as possible. Anything is an improvement over no weight loss plan at all.

Eat healthily:
If, after giving yourself enough time to transition to an intermittent fasting diet correctly and you still feel as though you are hungrier than you think you should be, you may want to consider the types of foods you are consuming and not just how many calories you are taking in each day. If you are eating a significant amount of processed foods, then you are likely not getting the level of nutrition that your body needs in a day, especially when you take the intermittent fasting into account. This means your body is burning through its available fuel faster than it should be. To counteract this development, merely add more healthy fats and lean protein to your diet. This should keep you feeling fuller

for extended periods of time and make intermittent fasting easier to stick to. Some good examples of foods you could add are things like almonds, cashews, macadamia nuts, coconut, olive and avocado oil for healthy fats and lean beef mince, chicken breast, eggs and fish such as salmon for protein.

Don't settle for the first plan you try:
The sheer variety of different intermittent fasting plans available means that, even if you find the first program you try easy to stick with, there might be a better one out there for you. Not trying multiple applications before you settle on one specific type can cause you to lose out on something that is even better. After all, if there isn't anything better out there for you, then you can always come back around to your first choice and pick up where you left off. If you don't try them all, you'll never know. Of course, if you don't think you can last the full length of time then there is no point in pushing yourself past your tolerance level. Be aware of your limitations and choose accordingly.

Drink more water:
While many people will naturally see this tip and assume that it means it is essential to stay hydrated. In reality, it is a command to drink at least a gallon of water every day. This will not only help you to feel full while fasting, but it will also ensure that your body continues to process toxins out of your system during the transitional phase when you are getting used to intermittent fasting.

During this time, your body will efficiently detoxify itself and rid itself of toxins as it adjusts to going without a full stomach all the time.

Additionally, this is good advice in general because 40 percent of all adults in the US are currently suffering from a mild state of dehydration without even knowing about it. This is amplified during a fasted state as your body doesn't have the tools to fight off the adverse effects of this as quickly as it otherwise would. Remember, if you are feeling thirsty then it is already too late.

Treat caffeine like a tool:
Especially during the early days when you are going to be looking for all the help you can get to help your body adjust in the intermittent fasting transition phase. You are going to want to take full advantage of the fact that caffeine is an appetite suppressant. A cup of black coffee or sparkling water every 4 hours should make the early weeks of your fast much more manageable. It is essential not to go crazy with the caffeine, however, especially if you are drinking something like diet soda as artificial sweeteners when consumed in bulk can have a wide variety of unintended consequences. For men, too much caffeine can also wreak havoc on the prostate as well so use it but be responsible and sensible with it. Another tip is never start your day with a coffee, after 6-8 hours of sleep you wake up dehydrated, your body is craving water and adding caffeine to your system before

you give it that water will only dehydrate you even more. I normally get in at least a 600ml bottle of water minimum prior to taking in caffeine.

Ideally, you are going to want to think of caffeine as a tool to help you get through the early, more difficult, part of the intermittent fasting transition. The goal should be to ultimately get your body used to your new dietary lifestyle without needing any such crutches to get you through your fasting periods. If you rely purely on caffeine alone then it can quickly become a habit of its own which is why you should feel free to use it as needed during the first month but then strive to curtail its usage down to a few cups per day. This may be easier said than done, and you may still feel hungry with it gone, but you will be glad you did in the long run. Another great benefit of having caffeine in a fasted state is that it amplifies your mental focus. You mental alertness will increase unbelievably and as a result you will become more productive in many other areas of your life such as work. This will help you keep busy and thus your mind off whatever hunger you are experiencing.

Keep busy:
It doesn't matter if you are just getting started with intermittent fasting or if you have been doing it for months, keeping busy is a great way to keep your mind, and your body occupied when hunger sets in so that you can more easily ignore it and complete your fast

successfully. Sitting around and thinking about the food that you will be eating when you break your fast is only going to make the time pass more slowly and leave you feeling hungrier as well.

Furthermore, you are going to want to make an effort to schedule all of your strenuous or difficult tasks either during the periods of time when you are free to eat, early on in a fast when you are still feeling somewhat full, or right at the end of your fast so that you can transition directly from the task to a beautiful, rewarding meal. Starting off a fast with unwanted duties might not be entirely pleasant, but holding off on those things for an extended period is only going to make them more challenging to complete in the long run when you have to dedicate more of your physical and mental energy to ignore your hunger.

Treat yourself:
When you first start fasting on a regular basis, you may want to build some rewards into your dietary plan to help ensure you remain motivated throughout the process. This means that at the end of the first week of fasting there is no real harm in splurging a little as long as you don't eat so much that you counteract all the hard work you have been doing. Remember, 3,500 calories is your target for one pound of fat loss per week so if you go over this amount then renew your drive by treating yourself to something that shows you appreciate all the hard work you are doing.

It is important not to feel guilty about these rewards, as this will defeat the purpose of having them in the first place. After all, you are making a very positive life change; you deserve a little something for dedicating yourself to a cause. Rather than feeling guilty about splurging a little, you will be better off remembering all of the meals that you have already skipped and how you are on your way to a better, healthier life.

Think about how much better off you already are and remind yourself that you are just getting started on a path that can help you live longer and feel better than you ever thought possible. Just be sure that you don't let one splurge turn into an entire day of splurging as falling back into bad behaviors never made anyone feel better in the long run.

Chapter 9: Common Fasting Mistakes and How to Avoid Them

At this point, I am more than a bit hopeful that you are ready to begin your intermittent fasting journey. But, before you start, I've listed some of the mistakes people make while fasting as well as ways you can avoid making them too.

1. Quitting before you give intermittent fasting a fighting chance:

It's a lifestyle! Yes - it's a challenging transition, but the potential rewards are AMAZING! I've read many stories of people who have fasted for two and half hours and called it quits. For Pete's sake, everyone can fast for at least 6 hours right out of the box. How do I know that? Because even the worst sleeper has had a "restful" 6 hours of sleep every once in a while.

(PS- have I mentioned that intermittent fasting could improve your sleep?)

One of the most visceral accounts of this "quitting out of the gate" mentality was a man who kept a journal about preparing for his first intermittent fast. I read with interest, as he parroted back his positive research findings, added up all the potential benefits, and ate his last meal in preparation for the BIG event. He wrote about the first couple of hours then stopped.... In the middle of a sentence! It was like, "I'm now twenty minutes into my second hour, and I have to say ..." That's all he wrote! I couldn't believe it, I felt sad for him. Sad for the missed opportunity. Sad that no one told him to take intermittent fasting at his own pace. Sad that he felt like he had failed again and probably "rewarded" himself by eating everything in the kitchen cupboard.

I'm going to ask you to please give intermittent fasting at least 30 days – one month to try it out and experience the changes it makes. Please don't limit yourself only to pounds lost. Take measurements every week around your stomach, chest, hips and legs. Take note of how your clothes fit, Journal how your sleep is and how your energy ebbs and flows. Write about your food choices and how you feel about the food you eat after a fasting period. Are you drawn to new and different foods than you have been in the past? Has the amount you eat changed? How often are you feeding during feeding periods? At the end of the 30 days, put it all together. I think you'll be pleasantly surprised that you did, and I'll be shocked if you're not!

2. Going the whole Hog on your first fast:

There is no humiliation in easing into intermittent

fasting. Take advantage of the many different sporadic fasting plans in existence and "date" a couple of them before making a significant commitment. You may find that several plans resonate more than others, and want to mix and match ideas or create your own hybrid version. Just remember the golden rules: No more than two 24-hour period fasts per week, and no two 24-hour fasts on consecutive days. For time restrictive plans, don't go more than 16 hours each day without feeding for the balance of the 24 hours.

Alternatively, design your gradual immersion schedule to settle yourself into intermittent fasting gracefully. You could accomplish this either by gradually extending the periods you fast or by decreasing progressively the hours you feed. The choice is yours as long as the goal of intermittent fasting remains authentic and the golden rules are adhered to.

3. Eating as much crappy food as you can!

So, you've been intermittently fasting religiously. You've got the timing down to the second, and you never cheat…during the fast. But when it's feeding time…BAM!!! All bets are off, and any indulgence is fair game. Okay. Deep breath. Let's have a reality check. Are you surprised you haven't lost much weight, or you don't feel so great, or you're experiencing a lot of gastric distress? It is a fantastic fact about human beings: we can take pretty much any "best practice" and warp it right out of recognition! It doesn't matter how good you are at the fasting part if you put bad gas in your tank at the end of the day. Here's a good rule of thumb if you're having a hard time coming to terms with the fact you can't eat like a drunken frat boy and lose weight by fasting intermittently: Just because you CAN (eat like a lumberjack) doesn't mean you SHOULD. Have your treats but make sure the bulk of your meals are made up of nutritious foods that will benefit your health so you get the absolute most out of your new lifestyle.

4. Going overboard with the "stimulants":

So, caffeine in the form of coffee and tea is allowed when you intermittently fast and that's a good thing. But, you know what they say about too much of a good thing... Remember the whole balance thing, so your pleasant morning coffee "euphoria" doesn't turn into a raging case of café nervosa! Too much caffeine will wreak havoc with your stomach and your nervous system. Drink coffee and tea mindfully, always keeping your tolerance levels in mind.

5. Fearing "the hunger":

Learn to recognize and come to terms with casual hunger. Know, with the growing assurance that comes when you get yourself use to intermittent fasting, that casual hunger is a passing thing. You know to understand that short-term fasting doesn't cause the body to "devour its own" muscle tissue or cause any other bodily harm. Don't let your mind play games with your intentions.

6. Overtraining:

While it's true that you might get away with intense workouts on fasting days, why take the chance of overextending or even injuring yourself? It is a simple fact that you will most likely feel better if you give your body a bit of a break on fasting days. Experts recommend taking a miss on long aerobic or cardio workouts on days when you are taking in less fuel. Try a more replenishing session of yoga, stretching or a weight training session with longer breaks in between sets instead, to prevent the discomfort and worry of dizziness or weakness.

7. Regarding intermittent feeding LESS does not equal MORE:

Be very careful not to start cutting down on your food intake to see if you can lose weight faster. Intermittent fasting is about moderation and balance between fasting and feeding. Don't tip this effective balance by cheating yourself out of the food you need to stay healthy. If you feel like this might be happening, seek medical help immediately!

8. Don't stalk the clock:

How ironic is it that the very same people who celebrate

the freedom and flexibility that intermittent fasting affords them often fall victim to endless and obsessive clock watching during fasting AND feeding periods. If you fall into this category, try and reinforce the flexibility of fasting by deregulating the exact times you eat during your feeding window. Experiment with snacking. Vary your mealtimes and make allowances for social interaction and special events. Be mindful about developing rigidity around eating. On the fasting side, if you start or end your fasting period a bit late from time to time or if your eating window happens to go slightly longer on a particular day don't let it ruin your day. Remember, with intermittent fasting every day offers the gift of another opportunity to get your health and wellness right!

9. Ignoring what your body is trying to tell you:

Intermittent fasting is only going to be good for you if your body accepts it. If you experience any symptoms besides the slight physical discomforts already discussed, you need to stop the fast immediately. This includes vomiting, fainting, shortness of breath, panic attacks or any unexpected and sudden sharp pain. If you don't experience relief soon after stopping the fast, seek immediate medical assistance

Chapter 10: DO's and DON'TS of Intermittent Fasting

Don't Overindulge Yourself

Do not overindulge yourself after the fast. Instead, begin a healthy routine by eating light meals 3-6 times daily. Avoid foods that aren't easily digestible. Little by little, include high fiber foods back into your meal plan and be careful when consuming alcohol if you do take it. Avoid overindulging in every aspect and limit yourself to a bottle of beer or a 5-ounce glass of wine.

Don't Forget to Keep Yourself Hydrated

It is essential to ensure that you drink enough water every day while fasting. How do you know if you're drinking enough water? Check your urine and see if it's light in color or yellowish. When the color is light, straw-colored or lemonade, then you are well hydrated, but if it's bright yellow or amber, you're dehydrated. Drink more water if your urine belongs to the latter class of color.

Do Inform Your Doctor

Before you begin fasting, ensure you seek out the advice of your doctor, especially, if you have health issues that relate to fasting. It also recommended that people without health issues keep their primary health care provider abreast of their plans.

Do Pay Attention to Signs and Symptoms

As stated there are side effects that come with fasting? This is why it is crucial to listen to your body and pay attention to signs that suggest you're pushing too hard or too fast. Watch out for symptoms like dizziness, weaknesses, heart palpitations and the likes and stop fasting immediately if you experience them! Don't be a hero and do away with anything that will put your well-being at risk.

Do Fit Your Fast into Your Plan

Have a thorough plan before fasting as you look to choose the most suitable day for you. Days during which you are stressed shouldn't be a fasting day. You can make your weekend your fasting days if you don't have much going on. If you do, pick two days a week, say Monday, as it's the beginning of the week and Thursday right before the weekend, you can then eat normally over the weekend.

Don't go Overboard with Your Last Supper

Avoid going overboard with your last food before a fast. It's advisable to consume foods containing lots of vegetables, healthy fat and lean protein. Fruits and legumes can also be taken as fruits provide you with natural sugar which can help calm your hormones. When you take in healthy meals before fasting, your body will be provided with a more slow-burning form of nutrition that will help carry you throughout your fasting period.

Do Prepare Your Mind, Body and Soul

It's essential to be emotionally and mentally prepared before you commence fasting. Have a deep thought about what you want to do, why you are doing it and how to achieve it. Make proper preparations after this and ensure you do away with foods or drinks that you shouldn't be taking during your fasted period to avoid temptation. If you're able to avoid these foods during this period, there's a high tendency that you may never retake them.

Do Make Sure You're Fit to Fast

Are you presently on prescription drugs, pregnant, diabetic, lactating or do you have underlying medical conditions? Then intermittent fasting is not for you. Do not fast if you belong to any of the above class to avoid unpredictable reactions. Instead of fasting, why not embrace the act of eating foods in their natural state and do away with any form of fatty, sugary, rich or highly processed foods? Consuming foods such as vegetables, fruits, and whole grains makes you healthier. Also, fasting is not ideal for people under the age of 18.

Do Take Your Vitamins

You need supplements to get most of the vitamins your body needs during fasting. This is especially true if you don't eat nutritious healthy foods during your eating window. To aid digestion during fasting, take vitamins in liquid form. During fasting, you'll be losing out on lots of vitamins and minerals you should have gotten from food. Do ensure you consult your doctor or health practitioner, to get the best supplement that will provide you with the total daily vitamins you need.

Do Find Fun Distractions

As mentioned previously while fasting, you need to engage in a couple of distracting activities to avoid hunger triggers. The fact that you're fasting doesn't mean you shouldn't have fun. You can go window shopping, sightseeing, strolling or do anything that interests you. Avoid meeting at a restaurant, going to the grocery store or other tempting activities that may force you into eating. Always have your goal of healthy weight loss in mind regardless of how daunting it may seem.

Do Get by With A Little Help from Your Friends

Getting through your fast may be difficult, causing you to appear irrational some times. To ease off, you can get a little help from your partner or friends that share the same idea with you. Contacting other fasters either offline or online is also a good idea. Join my private Facebook group **"effortless weight loss and functional strength"** and share your thoughts with me and others on the same journey as yourself, talk about your challenges and more. You can also keep a journal or record events about your daily activities. Doing this will help you keep up with your progress and devise means of getting better results when you know what you're doing wrong and putting those plans into action.

Don't Stress

Chilling can be calming and relieving but stressing yourself will raise your cortisol levels. When you stress yourself out either mentally or physically with certain types of exercises, more fat will be stored leading you in the opposite direction to where you want to be going. As a result achieving a significant weight loss goal may turn out to be impossible.

Paying close attention to these do's and don'ts will guarantee the desired result from your intermittent fasting plan.

Before you go

Just a quick reminder about my free report on the 8 food traps that can lead to failure and the 4 popular diet tips you should never follow. Web address below

www.vipfastingreport.com

Need a little extra support? Join my free Facebook accountability group and get full access to myself to help you along the way. I answer every question and am fully committed to your success.

Effortless weight loss and functional strength

Follow me on Instagram for more tips and videos at **effortless_weightloss**

Any questions, please email me at **michael.zollo@hotmail.com**

References

https://www.livestrong.com/slideshow/1008373-master-fast-dos-donts/

https://www.healthline.com/nutrition/6-ways-to-do-intermittent-fasting

https://www.healthline.com/health/how-to-exercise-safely-intermittent-fasting